DEJA REVIEW™

Histology and Cell Biology

NOTICE

Medicine is an ever-changing science. As new research and clinical experience broaden our knowledge, changes in treatment and drug therapy are required. The authors and the publisher of this work have checked with sources believed to be reliable in their efforts to provide information that is complete and generally in accord with the standards accepted at the time of publication. However, in view of the possibility of human error or changes in medical sciences, neither the authors nor the publisher nor any other party who has been involved in the preparation or publication of this work warrants that the information contained herein is in every respect accurate or complete, and they disclaim all responsibility for any errors or omissions or for the results obtained from use of the information contained in this work. Readers are encouraged to confirm the information contained herein with other sources. For example and in particular, readers are advised to check the product information sheet included in the package of each drug they plan to administer to be certain that the information contained in this work is accurate and that changes have not been made in the recommended dose or in the contraindications for administration. This recommendation is of particular importance in connection with new or infrequently used drugs.

DEJA REVIEW™
Histology and Cell Biology

Second Edition

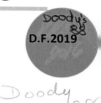

D.F.2019

Doody
score 88

Jae W. Song, MD, MS

Department of Surgery
University of Michigan Health Systems
Ann Arbor, Michigan

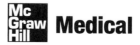 **Medical**

New York   Chicago   San Francisco   Lisbon   London   Madrid   Mexico City
Milan   New Delhi   San Juan   Seoul   Singapore   Sydney   Toronto

The *McGraw·Hill* Companies

Déjà Review™: Histology and Cell Biology, Second Edition

1 2 3 4 5 6 7 8 9 0   DOC/DOC   14 13 12 11 10

ISBN 978-0-07-162726-9
MHID 0-07-162726-X

This book was set in Palatino by Glyph International.

The editors were Kirsten Funk and Christine Diedrich.

The production supervisor was Catherine Saggese.

Project management was provided by Himi Anand, Glyph International.

RR Donnelley was printer and binder.

This book is printed on acid-free paper.

CIP data is on file with the Library of Congress.

McGraw-Hill books are available at special quantity discounts to use as premiums and sales promotions, or for use in corporate training programs. To contact a representative please e-mail us at bulksales@mcgraw-hill.com.

To my parents for their love, support, and sacrifices.
To my sister for being my muse.
To my friends and mentors for their inspiration.
—Jae W. Song, MD, MS

Contents

Faculty Reviewers

Jonathan F. Finks, MD
Assistant Professor of Surgery
University of Michigan Health System
Ann Arbor, Michigan

Page Wang, MD
Radiology Resident
University of Michigan Health System
Ann Arbor, Michigan

Robert M. Klein, PhD
Professor, Department of Anatomy
    and Cell Biology
University of Kansas Medical Center
School of Medicine
Kansas City, Kansas

Student Reviewers

Michael Allison
SUNY Downstate College of Medicine
Class of 2009

Stacy Cooper
SUNY Upstate Medical University
Class of 2008

Silke Heinisch
Temple University School of Medicine
MD/PhD Program
Class of 2010

David Scoville
University of Kansas School of Medicine
Class of 2011

Contributing Authors

Seema Kaura
General Surgery Resident
Westchester Medical Center
Valhalla, New York

Meera Meerkov
Medical Student
University of Michigan Health System
Ann Arbor, Michigan
Class of 2011

Megan H. Pesch
Medical Student
University of Michigan Medical School
Ann Arbor, Michigan
Class of 2011

Daniel J. Reiss
Medical Scientist Training Program
University of Michigan
Ann Arbor, Michigan

Preface

Thank you for using the *Deja Review: Histology and Cell Biology* book to assist you in your preparation for Step 1 of the United States Medical Licensing Exam (USMLE). We have worked diligently to bring you a concise and rigorous review of histology and cell biology to help you prepare for your Step 1 exam. This book is a compilation of all essential facts, organized into an easy-to-read Question and Answer format, with difficult concepts supplemented with figures and mnemonics. Furthermore, by combining clinical scenarios with fundamental principles, this review book encourages step-by-step logical problem solving skills, necessary for both good performance on the boards and success on the clinical wards. Considering the huge volume of information that you must synthesize in order to perform successfully as a clinician, we recommend the use of all the review books of this series to help you form that required foundation.

ORGANIZATION

The book is organized to review high-yield histology and cell biology concepts and tie in those concepts with clinical vignettes. The concepts found here cover the majority of topics as they are presented in a standard medical curriculum. In the histology section, special emphasis is placed on correlating histologic structure to physiologic function, and in the cell biology section, emphasis is placed on how cellular processes relate to medicine through their pharmacologic, physiologic, and pathologic roles. Each chapter ends with clinical correlates and vignettes exemplifying how basic histologic and cellular processes underlie disease.

Consistent with the other review books in this series, the Question and Answer format has several important advantages:

- It provides a rapid, straightforward way for you to assess your strengths and weaknesses.
- It offers numerous clinical vignettes that directly link fundamental histology and cell biology principles to clinical scenarios.
- It serves as a last minute review of up-to-date high-yield facts.
- It clarifies difficult concepts with numerous illustrations and tables.
- It is formatted to enable efficient reviewing of a large body of information.

HOW TO USE THIS BOOK

It is recommended that you use this book alongside a standard textbook to test your comprehension of the material. When preparing for exams, this book can be used as a quick, last minute review of high-yield facts. Please remember that while this book will be very useful for the USMLE Step 1 and for reviewing the fundamentals of medical science for your course exams, this review book should neither replace standard medical texts, lecture notes, nor substitute for sound clinical judgment. Rather, it is intended to help you understand difficult concepts, review high-yield topics, and provide you with a small portable book that is easy to use to quiz yourself and classmates on these concepts. A bookmark is included so that you can easily cover up the answers as you work through the questions in each chapter. The compact, condensed design of this book is conducive to studying on the go.

We hope you find this review book helpful during your preparation for the USMLE Step 1 exam and throughout medical school. Thank you for letting us help with your medical education!

Jae W. Song, MD, MS

Acknowledgments

The author would like to thank all the contributors, illustrators, and faculty and staff reviewers for their invaluable time and effort in contributing to this review book and making it a useful resource for all medical students. The author would like to recognize all faculty and staff at the University of Michigan Medical School, New York University School of Medicine, and Harvard Medical School for their endless commitment and dedication to educating medical students. Thank you to the students who used the first edition of this text to prepare for the boards and provided essential feedback necessary to write a higher-yield, comprehensive book. A special thanks to Kirsten Funk and Christine Diedrich at McGraw-Hill for their extraordinary patience and guidance at each step of the process to see this project through.

Finally, the author would like to acknowledge the following contributors for their work on the first edition:

Contributors
Jonathan Clarke
Brooke T. Davey
Gertjan Halbesma
Samar Saadat Hassouneh
Jimmie Honings
Alexander Iribarne
Ruchira M. Jha
Jane S. Kim
Catherine Yuan-Hsin Lau
Catherine Lee
Ankit I. Mehta
Kavita Menon
Benjamin S. Orozco

Kathleen Ruchalski
Sol Schulman
Seenu Susarla
Jeanie C. Yoon

Illustrators
Grzegorz Babiarz
Lukasz S. Babiarz
Alex M. Kotlyar
Pavel M. Kotlyar
Maki Ono
Christel Serirajwajra
Sharon J. Song

CHAPTER 1

Connective Tissue

What are the three major components of the extracellular matrix (ECM)?	1. **Protein/glycoprotein fibers** 2. **Ground substance** 3. **Water** (tissue fluid)
What are the specialized connective tissues of the body?	The **ABC**s: **a**dipose, **b**one, blood, and **c**artilage
Connective tissue elements arise primarily from which germ layer in the developing embryo?	Except for some connective tissues in the head, which arise from ectodermal neural crest cells (neuroectoderm), all other connective tissue elements have **mesodermal** origins.

GROUND SUBSTANCE

Ground substance is a complex mixture of space-filling glycoproteins and proteoglycans. How do glycoproteins differ from proteoglycans?	In general, they are opposites. **Glycoproteins** contain little sugar (branched carbohydrates) and extensive protein, whereas **proteoglycans** contain little protein and more sugar (linear polysaccharides formed from disaccharide repeats containing hexosamine).
What principal feature of proteoglycans underlies their barrier and adhesive functions?	The highly **negative charge**—since proteoglycans are polyanions, they bind cations and water creating electrostatic connections with other connective tissue elements. They also form a **bulky, yet highly viscous, fluid that prevents microbial penetration**.
Where are the proteoglycans distributed?	See Table 1.1

Table 1.1 Common Proteoglycans and Their Location

Proteoglycans	Location
Dermatan sulfate	Dermis, cartilage
Chondroitin sulfate	Near chondrocytes in bony and cartilaginous structures, cartilage
Keratan sulfate	Cornea, cartilage
Heparan sulfate	Basal laminae, cartilage

Which glycosaminoglycan is isolated primarily from vertebrate lung, liver, and mast cells, and is a potent anticoagulant that prevents the formation of stable blood clots?

Heparin is a negatively charged polymer of uronic acid and D-glucosamine that interacts with anti-thrombin III to deactivate the activated clotting factors IIa (thrombin), IXa, Xa, XIa, and XIIa and to block the clotting cascade.

What are the principal glycoproteins that function in cell adhesion to the ECM?

CLIF: Chondronectin, Laminin, Integrins (eg, laminin and fibronectin receptors), and Fibronectin

FIBERS

What are the three main types of connective tissue fibers and their protein constituents?

1. **Collagen fibers**: contain the glycoprotein collagen
2. **Reticular fibers**: contain the glycoprotein collagen
3. **Elastic fibers**: contain the protein elastin

COLLAGENS

What are the four main structurally and functionally distinct groups of collagens?

1. **Fibril-forming** collagens
2. **Fibril-associated** collagens
3. **Network-forming** collagens
4. **Anchoring** collagens

What natural and modified amino acids are principally found in collagen?

Natural amino acids—glycine and proline

Modified (hydroxylated) amino acids—hydroxylysine and hydroxyproline

What physical properties do collagen fibers impart to tissues?

Inelastic collagen fibers impart **strength and flexibility** to tissues.

Wound healing proceeds orderly from the acute inflammatory response, to parenchymal and connective tissue cell regeneration and finally to tissue remodeling and wound strengthening. What functions do the different collagen types have in wound healing?

Initially, **type III collagen** provides a temporary foundation for tissue regeneration; however, it is ultimately replaced by the **rigid, permanent type I collagen** for wound strength. Disordered type III hypercollagenization leads to excessive scarring or keloid formation.

RETICULAR FIBERS

What are reticular fibers?

Reticular fibers are **type III collagen** containing glycoproteins that create a flexible network in highly cellular organs that change shape and form (eg, liver, spleen, and hematopoietic organs).

What underlies the common staining characteristics of reticular fibers?

The **high carbohydrate content** causes reticular fibers to stain with silver salts and periodic acid-Schiff reagent (PAS).

ELASTIC FIBERS

What are the constituent fibers of elastic fibers?

Oxytalan and **elaunin** fibers

How do oxytalan and elaunin fibers form mature elastic fibers?

Oxytalan fibers = Glycoproteins + Fibrillin

Elaunin fibers = Oxytalan + Elastin

Elastic fibers = Elaunin + Elastin

What is the significance of the variable elastin composition of elastic fibers?

Oxytalan is elastin-poor, resulting in a stiffer fiber than **elaunin** and **elastic fibers,** which are elastin-rich. **Terminal** or **mature elastic fibers** have the greatest elasticity.

What are the natural and modified amino acids of elastin?

Natural amino acids—glycine and proline

Modified amino acids—desmosine and isodesmosine

What is the structural basis for the elasticity of the elastic fibers?

Covalently linked polylysine residues (desmosine and isodesmosine) that cross-link individual elastin fibers

What is the tissue distribution of the elastic fibers?

All fiber types are found in the skin; however, **oxytalan fibers** are found in the eyes, **elaunin fibers** are in sweat glands, and **elastic fibers** are in vessels.

CELLS

What do the resident and transient cells found within the loose (areolar) connective tissue include?

Resident cells include the adipocytes, macrophages, and tissue-specific blasts (eg, chondroblasts [cartilage], fibroblasts [connective tissue], osteoblasts [bone], and odontoblasts [dentin/teeth]).

Transient cells include leukocytes (neutrophils, eosinophils, basophils), lymphocytes, plasma cells, mast cells, and monocytes.

What general functions do these cells serve?

Tissue-specific blasts produce structural proteins and molecules. **Adipocytes** store energy and generate heat. **Tissue-specific leukocytes, lymphocytes,** and **plasma cells** are scouts of the immune system, providing surveillance and defending the body against incident microbes.

Fibroblasts are the most abundant connective tissue cell type. They are spindle-shaped cells with multiple projections, an oval nucleus, and acidophilic cytoplasm. What are the two types of fibroblasts and how do they differ from each other?

1. **Fibroblasts**
2. **Myofibroblasts**

Although both assist in wound healing by producing connective tissue fibers and ground substance, myofibroblasts use their actin-myosin contractile elements to close wounds (wound contracture).

In invasive ductal carcinoma of the breast, skin dimpling and nipple retraction often occur. What cell type is responsible for these findings?

Contractile myofibroblasts produce these phenomena by (1) contracting to initiate the retraction and (2) laying down type I collagen to maintain the retraction.

Tissue-specific macrophages are large monocyte-derived cells with granular appearing secondary lysosomes and a prominent eccentric kidney-shaped nucleus. What are five examples of tissue-specific macrophages?

1. **Kupffer cells**—liver
2. **Microglia**—central nervous system
3. **Osteoclasts**—bone
4. **Alveolar macrophages** ("dust cells")—lungs
5. **Langerhans cells**—skin

How does the reticuloendothelial system differ from the monocyte-macrophage system?

The **reticuloendothelial system comprises both the monocyte-macrophage** and **the lymphatic systems**.

What are multinuclear giant cells?

Macrophages that fail to digest a large foreign body and consequently coalesce with other macrophages forming a **cellular mass around the undigested foreign body.**

Two types of mast cells (mucosal and connective tissue mast cells) have been identified. The former cells reside in the alveoli and intestinal mucosa and contain granules of tryptase and chondroitin sulfate; the latter cells reside in the skin and intestinal submucosa and contain tryptase, chymase, carboxypeptidase, cathepsin G, and heparin. Based on their location and granule content, what are the functions of these two cell subtypes?

1. **Mucosal mast cells** are T-cell– and IgE-dependent and participate in immediate hypersensitivity reactions.
2. **Connective tissue mast cells** participate in wheal and flare reactions.

How do the two main populations of mast cells differ from each other?	1. **Granule content—connective tissue mast cells** contain heparin (anticoagulant) granules. 2. **Mucosal mast cells** contain inert chondroitin sulfate granules.
Immunohistochemical staining of mast cells can be achieved by searching for which receptor-ligand complex on the cell surface?	Mast cells contain specific **receptors for IgE**; consequently, staining for IgE and its receptor would yield numerous mast cells. The most effective stain for mast cells is **toluidine blue**, which provides a metachromatic reaction.
What significant light microscopic feature of mast cells provides evidence for a principal immune function of this cell type?	Prominent cytoplasmic granules containing **histamine, chemotaxis factors** (which aid in histamine release), **glycosaminoglycans**, and **proteases**—these molecules fuel immediate hypersensitivity reactions or anaphylaxis upon antigen reexposure.
From what cell type do the mast cell's surface IgE originate?	**Plasma cells**
In a hematoxylin and eosin-stained histologic section, how is a plasma cell differentiated from a mast cell?	**Plasma cells** have little cytoplasm and large, heterochromatin-containing nuclei that resemble clock faces, whereas **mast cells** have normal-appearing nuclei and abundant cytoplasmic granules.
Cromolyn and nedocromil are inhaled drugs used to treat asthma. They block the release of bronchoconstricting agents (ie, histamine) from mast cell granules. What is the mechanism of action of these drugs?	These **inhibitors of mast cell degranulation** turn off the phosphorylation- or calcium-dependent signal activated when antigen-complexed IgE binds its receptor on the mast cell's surface and tries to stimulate degranulation.

ADIPOSE TISSUE

What are the important distinguishing features of white and brown fat?	See Table 1.2
What histologic features underlie the principal functions of white fat versus brown fat?	See Table 1.3
What is the location of white fat and brown fat?	See Table 1.4

Table 1.2 Functional Differences Between White and Brown Fat

White Fat	Brown Fat
Energy storage and insulation Cushioning of vital organs Synthesis/secretion of hormones, cytokines, and growth factors (eg, leptin, angiotensinogen, and steroid hormones: testosterone, estrogen, glucocorticoid)	Ready source of lipid; when oxidized, it produces heat to warm the blood flowing through the brown fat.

Table 1.3 Histologic Differences Between White and Brown Fat

White Fat	Brown Fat
Large cells with a single fat droplet (unilocular)	Small cell with multiple fat droplets (multilocular)
Eccentric nucleus (signet ring appearance)	Centrally located nucleus
Yellow in color (carotenoids)	Brown in color (abundant mitochondria)
Basal lamina surrounding each cell	Sympathetic neuronal synapse on each cell

Table 1.4 Location of White and Brown Fat in Human Body

White Fat	Brown Fat
Connective tissue under the skin of abdomen, buttocks, axilla, and thigh	Large amounts in newborns to offset extensive heat loss due to high surface to mass ratio. Seen widely in body up to 10 years of age.
Greater omentum, mesentery, retroperitoneal space, and kidneys	Amount decreases as the body grows.
Acts as a cushion at the palms of hands and feet, beneath the visceral pericardium and the orbits around the eyeballs	Remains around the kidneys, adrenal glands, aorta, neck, and mediastinum.

Considering that "like dissolves like," what prevents cytoplasmic lipid droplets from diffusing through the plasma membrane of adipocytes and coalescing in the extracellular space?

Each fat cell membrane is reinforced by a **basal lamina**, and a **filamentous barrier** surrounds each lipid droplet preventing contact with the plasma membrane.

How is multilocular adipose tissue organized histologically?

Multilocular adipose tissue is organized into connective tissue delimited lobules of cell aggregates that run along dilated capillaries.

How does the adipocyte respond to epinephrine and glucagon during the starvation state?

During the starvation state, high epinephrine and glucagon levels (with respect to insulin) activate hormone-sensitive lipoprotein lipase and convert triglycerides to free fatty acids. **Profound, prolonged starvation leads to adipocyte atrophy.**

CONNECTIVE TISSUE TYPES

How does loose connective tissue differ from dense connective tissue?

Though both types contain all connective tissue elements, dense connective tissue has more collagen fibers and fewer cells than loose connective tissue.

What is the physiologic significance of the histologic difference between loose and dense connective tissue?

Loose connective tissue: insulation

Dense connective tissue: stress resistance

What two histologic patterns does dense connective tissue adopt?

1. A **regular pattern** due to the parallel alignment of collagen fibers
2. An **irregular pattern** due to the unaligned, three-dimensional collagen meshwork

How is elastic tissue different from elastic fibers?

Elastic tissue contains parallel elastic fiber arrays with collagen fibers and fibroblasts lying between these arrays.

How does reticular tissue differ from reticular fibers?

Reticular tissue is a spongy network of branched **reticular fibers** (type III collagen) and **ground substance** lined with reticular cells.

CLINICAL CORRELATES AND VIGNETTES

A 14 yo M w/ a h/o recurrent rectal prolapse in early childhood p/w fragile, easily bruised skin, joint laxity, and a heart murmur. What is the most likely diagnosis and what connective tissue defect causes this disorder?

Ehlers-Danlos Syndrome (EDS). The most common form is caused by a mutation in the gene encoding for type V collagen, which results in abnormal collagen synthesis. This leads to reduced tensile strength of connective tissue. This form of EDS follows an AD inheritance pattern.

A 20 yo M p/w a concave chest, a heart murmur and poor vision. He has a h/o dissecting aortic aneurysm in male relatives. What is the most likely connective tissue disorder and what type of connective tissues are affected?

Marfan syndrome is an AD disorder with a missense mutation in the *fibrillin-1* (*FBN-1*) gene on chromosome 15, resulting in the production of defective fibrillin. Common symptoms include lens dislocations, dissecting aortic aneurysms, cardiac valvular prolapse, joint hyperextensibility, long limbs, and tall stature.

A 25 yo F p/w a small hole in the superior pinna following an intentional piercing and subsequent removal of the earring 5 years ago. What characteristic of cartilage leads to the poor healing capabilities of this substance?

Mature cartilage has a limited capacity for repair and regeneration mostly due to its poor blood supply. Cartilage is devoid of blood vessels.

CHAPTER 2

Specialized Connective Tissues: Bone and Cartilage

What is cortical bone?

Forming nearly 80% of bone, **cortical bone is the dense outer layer** of bone composed of **layered, cylindrical collagen sheets (osteons)**. There are central (Haversian) vessels traversing the Haversian canals with radiating nutrient microvessels outlined by canaliculi within the bone. **Osteocytes** reside in lacunae lying between the calcified collagen sheets.

What is trabecular bone?

Forming 20% of bone, **trabecular bone is the spongy inner layer** of bone that forms the marrow space; it is composed of resorbed osteons and has poor vascularization.

How do cortical and trabecular bones differ histologically and functionally?

While no histologic differences exist between the two types of bone, **trabecular bone** has a high surface area to volume ratio, thus allowing it to be resorbed rapidly. By contrast, **cortical bone** has a low surface area to volume ratio and is resorbed slowly along the longitudinal axis.

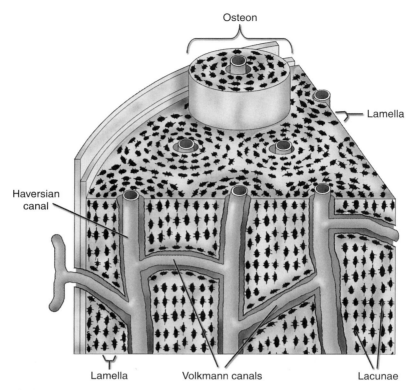

Figure 2.1   Cortical bone.

Osteoblasts are metabolically active, basophilic fibroblasts that line lacunae. How does this cell function in bone growth and remodeling?

Just remember, "**b**lasts **b**uild **b**one!" **Osteoblasts** secrete new bone matrix proteins for subsequent calcification and produce alkaline phosphatase leading to calcification.

What constitutes the connective tissue matrix of bone and lends to its hardness and inflexibility?

Fibril-forming, type I collagen and proteoglycans provide the organic scaffold onto which calcium hydroxyapatite is primarily deposited. Matrix vesicles play a key role in this process.

Osteoclasts are multinucleated giant cells derived from the monocyte-macrophage system. How does this cell function in bone growth and remodeling?

Just remember, "**c**lasts **c**hew **b**one!" Stimulated by parathyroid hormone (PTH) **osteoclasts resorb bone**, releasing Ca^{2+} into the circulation.

What ultrastructural feature of osteoclasts is responsible for its function?

Osteoclasts form sealed-off pits with the calcified bone matrix, which function as large "extracellular" lysosomes. Upon stimulation, the osteoclast cell membrane is stimulated to form folds called a "ruffled border" buried in the bone matrix. H^+ adenosine triphosphatases (H^+-ATPases) from endosomes are released into the extracellular space and function as secondary lysosomes acidifying the bone matrix leading to collagen degradation. **Urine pyridinoline**, a collagen breakdown product, is measured to assess the degree of bone resorption in patients.

Osteopetrosis is a rare condition where osteoclasts are defective and osteoblasts function unopposed. What are the clinical consequences of excessive bone formation?

In **osteopetrosis**, overgrowth of trabecular bone crowds out the bone marrow **leading to anemia and splenomegaly due to extramedullary hematopoiesis**. In the long term, nerve compression results from cortical bone overgrowth leading to the narrowing of neural foramina.

By what process does hyaline cartilage (precursor of bone) develop into bone?

Endochondral ossification is involved in the formation of the bones of the axial skeleton that bear weight and in the natural healing of bone fractures.

What is the name of the process by which bone formation results from the differentiation of mesenchymal cells into osteoblasts?

Intramembranous ossification is involved in the formation of the flat bones of the skull and face, mandible, and clavicle.

Epiphyseal cartilage at the ends of bones can be divided into five zones: hyalinized resting zone, the proliferative zone, the hypertrophic cartilage zone with enlarged chondrocytes, the calcified cartilage zone, and the zone of ossification containing hematopoietic and osteogenic stem cells. What is this structure, and how does it function in bone growth?

The regions of active chondrocyte proliferation found at the ends of long bones are called **epiphyses**. Stimulation by **growth hormone–generated IGF-1** increases cartilage and bone matrix formation at open epiphyseal plates. Conversely, **estrogens** arrest chondrocyte proliferation enabling epiphyseal closure.

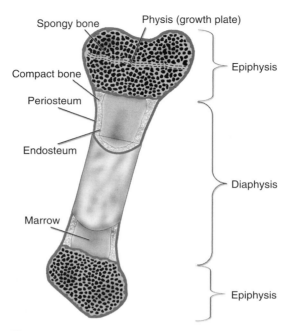

Figure 2.2   General long bone organization.

Synostotic, syndesmotic, and synchondrotic joints contain bone, dense connective tissue, and hyaline cartilage, respectively. However, diarthrotic joints contain a dense connective tissue capsule lined with fibroblasts and macrophages (synovium) and surrounds two apposing hyaline cartilage sheets. What is the functional difference between synovial and non-synovial joints?

Because of the presence of a synovium, which produces viscous, hyaluronic acid-rich, synovial fluid, **only diarthrotic joints exhibit free and frictionless movement**.

CARTILAGE

Cartilage contains islands of cells immediately surrounded by an intensely basophilic extracellular matrix. What are the three types of cartilage?

1. Hyaline cartilage
2. Elastic cartilage
3. Fibrocartilage

How do the three types of cartilage differ from each other?	The three types of cartilage are distinguished by the proportions of proteoglycans, glycosaminoglycans, and collagen and elastic fibers. **Fibrocartilage** contains abundant type I collagen, **hyaline cartilage** contains type II collagen, and **elastic cartilage** contains both type II collagen and elastic fibers.
Since cartilage is avascular, denervated, and without lymphatic drainage, how do chondrocytes acquire nutrients?	By **simple diffusion** from blood vessels within the dense perichondrium
What facilitates the principal shock absorptive function of cartilage?	The **test-tube brush–shaped proteoglycan aggregates** and **water** produce the shock absorptive bulk of articular cartilage.
What is the anatomic distribution of the three types of cartilage?	1. **Hyaline cartilage**—articular surfaces and large airways 2. **Elastic cartilage**—ears and airways 3. **Fibrocartilage**—intervertebral disks

CLINICAL CORRELATES AND VIGNETTES

A 2 yo F adopted from Haiti two weeks ago p/w bowing of legs. What is the name and cause of her condition?

Rickets. This condition is caused by decreased vitamin D synthesis, absorption, metabolism, or dietary deficiency. It results in **derangement of endochondral ossification** leading to loss of structural rigidity of developing bones and skeletal deformities.

A 25 yo M p/w a broken tibia following a skateboarding accident. Plain film demonstrates a wedge-shaped area of radiolucency in the femur. What histological changes would be common in this condition?

Paget disease. Disorder is characterized by rapid bone turnover with excessive bone resorption and formation leading to disorganized bone structure, called a **mosaic pattern of lamellar bone**. The wedge-shaped area of radiolucency is also known as the "blade of grass" sign. It indicates active Paget disease. Histologic and cellular abnormalities are noted in the morphology and activity of osteoblasts and osteoclasts, respectively.

A 61 yo F p/w a fractured proximal femur following a fall while walking on ice. What is the diagnosis this woman likely carries and what changes are seen in the osteoclast/osteoblast activity?

Osteoporosis. This condition is often seen in postmenopausal women. **Osteoblasts** demonstrate reduced replicative and biosynthetic potential in the elderly, while **osteoclast** activity increases.

CHAPTER 3

Blood

What are the two major components of blood?

1. **Cellular phase** (ie, formed elements)
2. The **Liquid phase or plasma**

Blood is often included as a connective tissue because it consists of cells and matrix (plasma).

Formed elements consist of what three cell types?

1. Erythrocytes or red blood cells (RBCs)
2. Leukocytes or white blood cells (WBCs)
3. Thrombocytes or platelets

Arrange the formed elements in order of decreasing size.

leukocytes > erythrocytes > thrombocytes

What is it called when erythrocytes appear as large as some leukocytes on a smear?

Macrocytosis—when present in anemia, macrocytosis is usually **caused by folic acid** or **vitamin B_{12} deficiency.**

What is it called when erythrocytes appear to be as small as some platelets on a smear?

Microcytosis—when present in anemia, microcytosis is commonly **caused by iron deficiency** and **severe thalassemia.**

What are the constituents of plasma?

1. Water (90%)
2. Proteins (7%)
3. Inorganic ions (less than 1%; eg, Na^+, K^+, Cl^-, and PO_4^{3-})
4. Small molecules (2%; eg, amino acids, carbohydrates, vitamins, and hormones)

What is the difference between plasma and serum?

Serum = Plasma − fibrin clot components

What are major protein constituents of plasma?

1. Albumin
2. α-Globulins (eg, hormone and heavy metal-binding globulins)
3. β-Globulins (eg, transferrin and plasminogen)
4. Gamma globulins (eg, immunoglobulins)
5. Fibrinogen and coagulation factors
6. Complement proteins, lipoproteins
7. Electrolytes (eg, Na^+, Cl^-)

What is the most abundant cell type found on a blood smear?

RBCs

Can a change in erythrocyte count be visualized on a blood smear?

No. However, a significant increase or decrease in leukocytes or platelets can be detected on a blood smear. **Excess leukocytes** can occur in acute or chronic, myelocytic or lymphocytic leukemia, whereas **decreased lymphocytes** can indicate marrow failure.

ERYTHROCYTES

RBCs are anucleate biconcave bags of hemoglobin. Name the proteins involved in maintaining the biconcavity.

Remember, "**SAAB!**"

Spectrin, Actin, Ankyrin, and Band-3

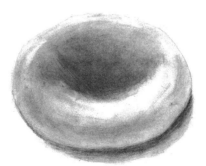

Figure 3.1   Erythrocyte.

In addition to the nucleus, which other organelles are absent from RBCs?

All organelles are missing from mature erythrocytes.

What state is indicated by pale RBCs with increased central clearing?

Hypochromia, due to a decrease in the mean cellular hemoglobin content; this state usually **occurs in severe iron deficiency anemia**.

How do reticulocytes differ from mature RBCs?

Reticulocytes are **larger** than mature RBCs; they contain **ribosomes, mitochondria,** and **cytoplasmic granules.**

What is the principal function of RBCs?

RBCs contain hemoglobin, which **delivers oxygen** to body tissues. Under normal conditions, CO binds hemoglobin to form carboxyhemoglobin more avidly than O_2 and CO_2, which bind hemoglobin to form carbaminohemoglobin. When greater than 70% of hemoglobin contains CO, death occurs rapidly (CO poisoning).

LEUKOCYTES

What are the two main types of leukocytes?

1. **Granulocytes**
2. **Agranulocytes**

Distinction is based on the leukocyte's nuclear shape and type of cytoplasmic granule.

Granulocytes have multilobular nuclei and abundant cytoplasmic (specific and azurophilic) granules. Azurophilic granules (or lysosomes) stain purple, whereas specific granules stain red, white (neutral), or blue based on their protein and macromolecular composition. What functions are associated with these histologic features?

The granules contain proinflammatory cytokines and chemokines, microbicidal proteins, proteases, and metalloproteases, in addition to substances that promote allergic reactions. Those substances **promote acute inflammation, allergic responses**, and **microbial killing.**

Which cells constitute the granulocyte class?

All the "phils": **neutrophils, eosinophils,** and **basophils.**

NEUTROPHILS

Making up 60% to 70% of peripheral blood leukocytes, neutrophils are the most abundant peripheral blood granulocyte. How do neutrophils typically look under a microscope (three features)?

1. **Multilobular nucleus** connected by slender threads and hence called polymorphonuclear leukocytes (PMNs)
2. **Neutral** (ie, unstained) **granules**
3. **Azurophilic granules**

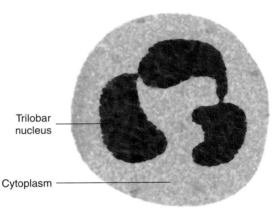

Trilobar
nucleus

Cytoplasm

Figure 3.2   Neutrophil.

What feature of immature neutrophils (or bands) easily distinguishes them from mature neutrophils?

Bands have horseshoe-shaped nuclei, whereas **PMNs** have multilobular nuclei connected by thin chromatin threads.

What adjective describes a neutrophil that has six or more nuclear lobules?

Hypersegmented—this appearance usually indicates old cell age or pathology, like vitamin B_{12} or folate deficiency.

Neutrophilic granules contain a host of proteins and macromolecules, including membrane-bound nicotinamide adenine dinucleotide phosphate (NADPH) oxidase, myeloperoxidase, α-defensins, elastase, and two metalloproteinases. What roles do these substances play in neutrophil function?

Phagocytosis of invading bacteria triggers neutrophilic granule release into the phagocytic vacuole and the extracellular space. In the vacuole, antimicrobial defensins and acidic oxidant–producing myeloperoxidase assist the O_2^- and H_2O_2 produced by NADPH oxidase and superoxide dismutase in killing bacteria. Meanwhile, in the extracellular space, the metalloproteinases and elastases degrade collagen and elastin, thus enabling the oxidizing bactericidal agents to produce a killing zone around the neutrophil.

EOSINOPHILS

Though eosinophils make up 5% of the circulating leukocytes, they are easily identified on a blood smear. What are the two prominent histologic features of an eosinophil?

1. Bilobed nucleus
2. Large, bright orange to red specific granules

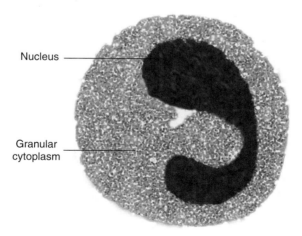

Nucleus

Granular cytoplasm

Figure 3.3   Eosinophil.

What are the major functions of eosinophils?

1. Have phagocytic capabilities
2. Defend against parasitic infections
3. Increase tissue damage in the "late phase" of immediate hypersensitivity reactions
4. Limit the severity of allergic reactions by secreting histaminase, which degrades histamine

Eosinophilic granules contain major basic protein, eosinophil cationic protein, eosinophil-derived neurotoxin, lysophospholipase, acid hydrolases, and peroxidase. What roles do these substances play in eosinophil function?

Recruited and stimulated by interleukins 4 and 5 (IL-4 and 5), respectively, eosinophils respond to IgE-coated parasites by binding the IgE and discharging their granule contents onto the opsonized organism. **These proteins all work to degrade the parasitic cell wall effectively killing the organism.**

A clinically significant increase in the number of eosinophils can signal specific conditions, like parasitic infection, systemic allergic disorder, a drug reaction, dermatitis, and even B- and T-cell lymphomas. What is a major clinical consequence of profound chronic eosinophilia?

Major basic protein and eosinophil cationic protein are potent host cytotoxins. Prolonged eosinophilia produces **profound tissue damage leading to an irreversible, restrictive endomyocardial fibrosis and in extreme cases widespread organ dysfunction.**

BASOPHILS

What are the key histologic features of basophils?

Basophils are identified by **their large, deep purple specific granules that obscure the trilobular nuclei.** An increased number of basophils in a smear may indicate the presence of a myeloproliferative disorder, like chronic myelogenous leukemia.

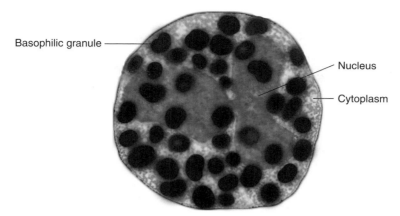

Basophilic granule

Nucleus

Cytoplasm

Figure 3.4   Basophil.

What accounts for the basophilia of the granules?

Heparin—basophilic granules contain histamine, 5-hydroxytryptamine, and sulfated proteoglycans.

Basophils closely resemble but are distinct from which immune cells found predominantly in tissues other than blood?

Mast cells—basophils and mast cells actually have different cell origins within the bone marrow; however, they perform similar functions in their respective compartments. Basophils circulate in the blood whereas mast cells are found in mucosae and connective tissue.

What is the principal function of a basophil?

Basophils function in immediate hypersensitivity reactions—antigen- and IgE-mediated receptor cross-linking and activation trigger the release of histamine and other inflammatory mediators. This release drives the development of urticaria, rhinitis, and anaphylactic shock.

Agranulocytes have round, occasionally clefted nuclei, and mildly imperceptible azurophilic granules. Which cells are agranulocytes?

Lymphocytes and **monocytes**.

LYMPHOCYTES

What are the four types of lymphocytes?

1. **B lymphocytes** (B-cells, plasma cells, and memory B-cells)
2. **T lymphocytes** (helper, cytotoxic, suppressor, and memory T-cells)
3. **Natural killer (NK) cells**
4. **Null cells**

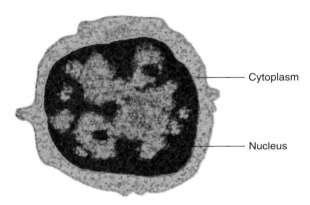

Cytoplasm

Nucleus

Figure 3.5   Reactive lymphocyte.

Lymphocytes constitute 20% to 25% of agranulocytes and may be small, medium, or large in size. Small lymphocytes have an intensely stained spherical nucleus and a scant cytoplasmic rim. Larger lymphocytes have more abundant cytoplasm, which may contain few granules. How are lymphocytes differentiated from each other by light microscopy?

Lymphocyte subtypes are histologically indistinguishable from one another; however, **cell surface markers facilitate immunocytochemical differentiation.**

What are the cell surface markers found on the various lymphocytes?

1. **T-cell**—T-cell receptor, CD1 to CD8.
2. **B-cell**—B-cell receptor, CD10, CD19 to CD23.
3. **NK cells**—CD16 and CD56.
4. **Null cell**—This catch-all group has characteristics of neither major class.

Lymphocytes vary from 9 to 14 μm in diameter. What does variable lymphocyte size indicate about its function?

Size indicates the degree of immunologic activation. A small lymphocyte, whether a B-cell or T-cell, becomes a large lymphocyte as it is stimulated to proliferate.

In what three ways do lymphocytes differ from granulocytes?

1. Lymphocytes have no granules.
2. Lymphocytes have single round, not multilobular, nuclei.
3. Lymphocytes have small cytoplasmic rims, not abundant cytoplasm.

What are plasma cells?

Plasma cells are the **terminally differentiated product of B-cell activation that produces a specific type of antibody**. They do not circulate in the blood under normal conditions.

What are the major functions of B-and T-lymphocytes?

B-and T-lymphocytes function in **acquired immunity**. B-cells produce antibodies and are critical in **humoral immunity**; CD8$^+$ cytotoxic T-cells are key players in **cell-mediated immunity**. CD4$^+$ helper T-cells coordinate the immune response by driving it toward either cell-mediated immunity with Th1 cells using IL-2 and interferon-γ or humoral immunity with Th2 cells using IL-4 and 5.

What are the principal functions of NK cells?

Induced and activated by IL-12 and 15, respectively, **NK cells lyse virally infected, IgG-coated, or major histocompatibility complex class I (MHC-I)–deficient cells using a host of specialty proteins**. Activated NK cells punch holes in target cells with perforins, then induce apoptosis with granzymes or kill intracellular microbes with granulysin. Afterward, with interferon-γ, NK cells recruit macrophages to phagocytose the killed cells.

MONOCYTES

What are the three histologic features of monocytes?	1. Eccentric, **kidney-shaped nuclei** 2. **Basophilic cytoplasm** 3. Fine **azurophilic granules**

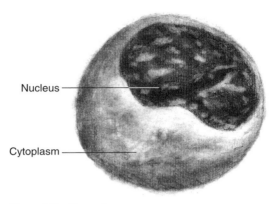

Nucleus

Cytoplasm

Figure 3.6   Monocyte.

Blood monocytes migrate into the tissues and turn into what cell type?	Macrophages
What are the principal functions of macrophages?	Attracted by chemokines, activated macrophages **migrate toward a stimulus and phagocytose foreign organisms or damaged cells**. These cells also function as antigen presenting cells in adaptive immunity by presenting antigens to B- and T-lymphocytes.

PLATELETS

What are the major histologic features of platelets?

1. **Granulomere**—central, purple, granulated zone
2. **Anucleate cell fragments**
3. **Hyalomere**—peripheral, blue-staining zone

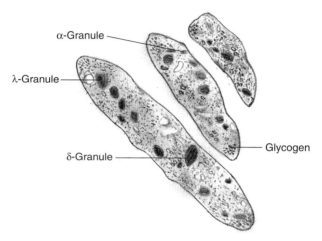

α-Granule

λ-Granule

δ-Granule

Glycogen

Figure 3.7   Platelets.

What are the three proteins found within the hyalomere that assist in contraction and degranulation?

1. **Microtubule** bundles provide structure and the tracks for degranulation.
2. **Actin** provides the mechanism for platelet contraction upon activation.
3. **Myosin** also provides the mechanism for platelet contraction upon activation.

What are the main functions of platelets?

1. Promote blood clotting
2. Repair gaps in blood vessel walls

HEMATOPOIESIS

What cells are derived from the lymphoid lineage of cells?

1. B-lymphocytes
2. T-lymphocytes
3. NK cells
4. Null cells

What cells are derived from the myeloid cell line?

1. Granular leukocytes
2. Monocytes
3. Megakaryocytes

On gross examination, what are the two types of bone marrow?

1. **Red marrow**: predominance of hematopoietic elements. Active and produces cellular blood components.
2. **Yellow marrow**: predominance of adipocytes. Inactive and infiltrated with fat.

What are the three principal histologic components of red bone marrow?

1. Sinusoidal capillaries
2. Hematopoietic cords
3. Stroma (collagens I and III, reticular fibers and cells, hematopoietic cells, and macrophages)

Among the blood cells, which series can be readily discerned by microscopic examination of the bone marrow?

Just remember, "MEG"— megakaryocytic, erythrocytic, and granulocytic

MEGAKARYOCYTOPOIESIS

What two cells comprise the megakaryocytic series?

1. **Megakaryoblasts**
2. **Megakaryocytes**

How are megakaryoblasts differentiated from megakaryocytes (four features)?

1. Megakaryocytes are three times **larger**—these are the largest cells in the bone marrow.
2. They have **irregularly lobulated**, rather than ovoid or kidney-shaped, **nuclei**.
3. They are **not multinucleoliated**.
4. They have a **granulated** rather than homogeneous, basophilic **cytoplasm**.

ERYTHROPOIESIS

In order, what are the six cells of the erythroid series?

Just remember, "In life, either **pro**duce or be **pore**"—**pro**erythroblasts, **b**asophilic, **p**olychromatophilic, and **o**rthochromatophilic erythroblasts, **r**eticulocytes, and **e**rythrocytes.

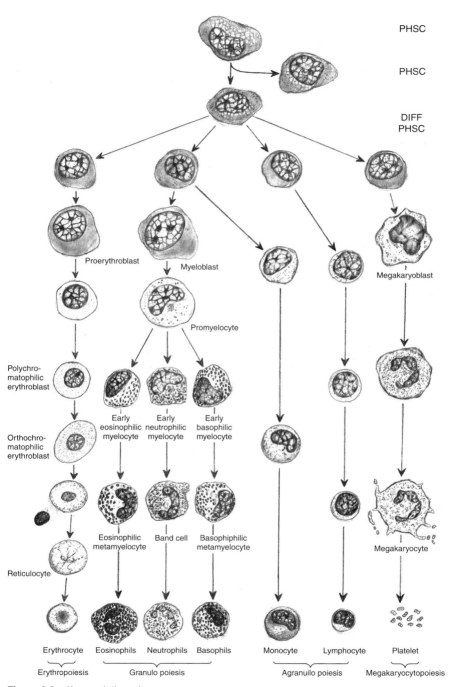

Figure 3.8   Hemopoietic series.

What are the prominent histologic features of each cell in the erythroid line?

Proerythroblasts (four features)

1. Basophilia (due to polyribosomes)
2. Large cell
3. Lacy chromatin
4. Prominent nucleolus

Basophilic erythroblasts (three features)

1. Basophilia (due to polyribosomes)
2. Condensed nucleus
3. Absent nucleolus

Polychromatophilic erythroblasts (two features)

1. Polychromatophilic (due to acidophilic hemoglobin and basophilic ribosomes)
2. Condensed nucleus

Orthochromatophilic erythroblasts (two features)

1. Acidophilia (due to hemoglobin)
2. Condensed nucleus

Reticulocyte (two features)

1. Anucleate
2. Lacy ribosomal RNA network visualized by brilliant cresyl blue

Erythrocyte

Anucleate, biconcave disks

GRANULOPOIESIS

What are the five cells of the granulocytic series, in order?

(See Figure 3.8)

1. Myeloblast
2. Promyelocyte
3. Neutrophilic (basophilic or eosinophilic) myelocyte
4. Band
5. Mature granulocyte

How is the major branch point in the three types of granulocytes recognized histologically?

By the development and expansion of specific granules—at this branch point, a common promyelocyte gives rise to neutrophilic, basophilic, and eosinophilic myelocytes.

What are the key histologic features of the cells of the granulocytic series?

Myeloblast—distributed chromatin and prominent nucleoli

Promyelocyte—basophilic cytoplasm and azurophilic (lysosomal) granules

Eosino-, neutro-, or basophilic myelocyte—red, neutral (white), or blue specific granules condensed nucleus

Band—horseshoe-shaped nucleus, specific granules

Mature granulocyte—chromatin thread–connected multilobar nucleus and specifically colored granules

AGRANULOPOIESIS

Why is one unable to differentiate the cells of the monocytic and lymphocytic series on microscopic examination of the bone marrow?

(See Figure 3.8)

No specific granules and **nondescript nuclei**

How are lymphocyte precursors differentiated?

Through **cell surface receptor–based immunocytochemical or cell-sorting methods using fluorescent flow cytometry** with appropriate cell surface markers

CLINICAL CORRELATES AND VIGNETTES

3 yo M p/w yellowing of skin and eyes following an infection with Parvovirus B19 (fifth disease). What is the most likely diagnosis, and what changes in RBC shape would be seen on blood smear?

Hereditary Spherocytosis (HS). Mutations weaken the interactions of **S**pectrin, **A**ctin, **A**nkyrin, and **B**and-3 (SAAB), resulting in a spherical RBC shape. On blood smear, spherocytes appear abnormally small, hyperchromic, and lack central zone of pallor. Symptoms commonly present following aplastic crisis triggered by an acute parvovirus infection.

65 yo M p/w fatigue, pale skin, and recent history of hematochezia. What RBC changes would you expect to see on a blood smear?

Microcytic and **hypochromic RBCs.** RBCs would appear smaller and paler when observed by a blood smear due to anemia.

CHAPTER 4

Muscle

SKELETAL MUSCLE

What features of skeletal muscle facilitate its identification by light microscopy?

1. **Striations**, which represent the different bands and zones of the **sarcomere**
2. **Multinucleated cells** with **peripherally located nuclei**

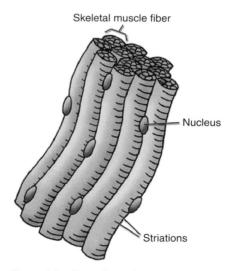

Skeletal muscle fiber

Nucleus

Striations

Figure 4.1 Skeletal muscle fascicle.

How is skeletal muscle organized?

The whole muscle, considered a bundle of fascicles, is surrounded by the **epimysium; perimysium** surrounds the individual fascicles (bundle of fibers). **Endomysium**, a basement and cell membrane, surrounds each muscle fiber (skeletal myocyte), which contains parallel filamentous contractile protein bundles, called **myofibrils**.

What structure, critical to skeletal muscle tone and contraction, runs and branches within the perimysial connective tissue?

Anterior horn cells in the spinal cord send motor nerve axons, which synapse on skeletal myocytes forming a **neuromuscular junction** (NMJ). At the NMJ, contraction is initiated when the myocyte membrane depolarizes and transmits that depolarization into the cell by **T-tubules**.

What muscle structure is responsible for force transmission throughout the contracting muscle?

The connective tissue capsules and septae formed by the **epi-, peri-,** and **endomysium** transmit force throughout the contracting muscle.

What protein complex, found within the muscle cell, is responsible for transmitting the force generated by contraction to the cell surface?

The **dystrophin glycoprotein complex** contains cytoplasmic and transmembrane proteins. These structures function in contractile force transmission to the cell surface and provide structural support to the myofibril. Congenital defects in this complex cause many of the **muscular dystrophies**, including **Duchenne** and **Becker muscular dystrophies**.

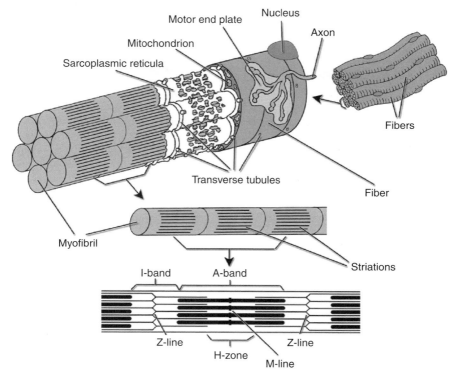

Figure 4.2 Muscle fiber and sarcomere.

The sarcomere is a repeating contractile unit of myofibrils, bound along their length by Z-bands. Name the zones of a sarcomere beginning with the M-line and ending with the Z-band.

Remember, **M**uscles **H**ave **A**lternating **I**nternal **Z**ones—M-line, H-band, A-band, I-band, and Z-band.

What zone of the sarcomere is responsible for force generation during muscle contraction?

The **A-band** or the region of **thick** and **thin filament** overlap within the **sarcomere** generates the force during muscle contraction.

Which bands shorten during skeletal muscle contraction?

I- and **H-bands**

Does either the thick or thin filament shorten significantly during muscle contraction?

No. According to the sliding filament model, muscle contraction is achieved by altering the relative positions of thick and thin filaments bringing adjacent Z-bands closer together without changing the length of the filaments themselves.

At the level of the sarcomere, what is the difference between isometric and isotonic contractions?

Isotonic contractions: thick and thin filaments slide along each other, shortening the length of the sarcomere and producing movement.

Isometric contractions: thick and thin filaments bind each other, but the sarcomeres do not change length—only tension is produced.

Skeletal muscle has at least two important functions—it contracts to enable movement, and it participates in metabolism by serving as a protein repository for metabolic needs. What physiologic process provides evidence for this metabolic role of muscle?

Skeletal myocytes degrade contractile proteins and become smaller in size (atrophy) in patients with poor nutrition. These patients appear thin and wasted.

During muscle breakdown due to ischemia and infarction, muscle proteins are released into the blood stream. To provide evidence for ongoing muscle breakdown, laboratory tests have been designed to detect these proteins. What clinically significant proteins are found in the following structures:

  M-line?

Creatine kinase

  H-band?

Myosin

  A-band?

Thick and overlapping thin filaments

  I-band?

Nonoverlapping thin filaments

What are the protein components of the thick and thin filaments?

Thin filaments—actin, tropomyosin, and the troponins (TnC, TnI, and TnT)

Thick filaments—myosin

What are the functions of the troponins and tropomyosin?

TnC: binds the calcium that initiates contraction

TnI: binds actin and inhibits actin-myosin interactions

TnT: binds other troponin components to tropomyosin

Tropomyosin: covers myosin-binding sites on actin filaments preventing actin-myosin interactions

What proteins, found at the Z-band, work to maintain the structural integrity of the sarcomere?

α-Actinin or **nebulin**: anchors thin filaments to the Z-band

Titin: provides the sarcomere with scaffolding, elasticity, and protection against overstretching by connecting the Z-band to the M-line

Desmin: ties adjacent sarcomeres together, while binding the Z-band to the plasma membrane

What are T-tubules?

A network of channels that are continuous with the plasma membrane and encircle the sarcomere at the junction of the A- and I-bands.

What are terminal cisternae?

Specialized Ca^{2+} storage and release depots located at the ends of the sarcoplasmic reticulum (SR)

Excitation-contraction coupling is the process whereby muscle fiber depolarization stimulates muscle contraction. What structures within the muscle fiber facilitate this process?

T-tubules and the **SR** work together to enable excitation-contraction coupling. T-tubules transmit the action potential rapidly from the cell membrane to all myofibrils; that action potential triggers the release of Ca^{2+} from terminal cisternae enabling contraction.

What small, mononuclear, fusiform cell population situated beneath the basement membrane would be depleted in a disease of continued muscle breakdown such as Duchenne or Becker muscular dystrophy?

The **regenerative cells** for skeletal muscle (**satellite cells**) would become depleted. These cells provide nuclei to skeletal muscle during hypertrophy and they synthesize new muscle after myocyte injury.

Rigor is a condition where muscle has stopped contracting and developed a rigid state. How does a rise in intracellular $[Ca^{2+}]$ and depletion of ATP result in muscular rigor?

Intracellular Ca^{2+} interacts with **troponin** causing tropomyosin to expose the myosin-binding site on thin filaments. Once myosin heads form cross bridges with thin filaments, the myosin heads can only dissociate in the presence of ATP. In the absence of ATP, myosin heads remain bound and muscular rigor results.

What are the differences between types I and II muscle fibers?

Type I—slow twitch; high oxidative phosphorylation; fat metabolizing; red macroscopically because of high myoglobin and mitochondrial cytochromes. They contract slowly, but are capable of repeated or continuous contraction. The mnemonic **"ONE SLOW RED OX"** is useful to help remember the characteristics of this fiber type.

Type II—fast twitch; low in oxidative activity; high substrate level phosphorylation; high glycolytic activity; white macroscopically. They are capable of rapid contraction but cannot maintain repeated contraction indefinitely. The mnemonic **"TWO FAST WHITE SUGAR"** helps recall these features.

What cellular and histologic features differ in muscles with grossly different functions such as the postural muscles of the back and the extrinsic muscles of the eye?

Postural muscles perform gross, strong, sustained contractions and are thus arranged in large motor units containing hundreds of slow-twitch fibers that are rich in myoglobin and mitochondria. In contrast, the extrinsic eye muscles perform rapid, precise movements and thus contain fast-twitch, glycolytic fibers in small motor units containing less than 10 fibers.

How does denervated skeletal muscle differ from denervated cardiac muscle?

Denervated skeletal muscle becomes hypersensitive to circulating acetylcholine and exhibits fine, irregular contractions (fibrillations). By contrast, since cardiac muscle does not require innervation for contraction, it neither atrophies nor experiences **acetylcholine hypersensitivity** and fibrillations upon denervation.

What is the difference between α- and γ-motor neurons?

α-Motor neurons: innervate extrafusal myofibers

γ-Motor neurons: innervate intrafusal (regulatory) myofibers

Nuclear bag and nuclear chain fibers are fusiform skeletal myocytes containing either a central, large aggregation (bag) of nuclei or a row (chain) of central nuclei extending the length of the muscle. What is the function of nuclear bag and chain fibers?

Nuclear bag and **chain fibers** are intrafusal muscle fibers composing part of the muscle spindle. **Muscle spindles** are mechanoreceptors that sense muscle length, tension, or stretch and generate a reflex response.

Considering the function of nuclear bag and chain fibers, how are they innervated?

These contractile receptors have both motor and sensory innervation. Nuclear bag fibers receive both β- and γ-motor innervation, whereas nuclear chain fibers receive only γ-motor innervation. Likewise, nuclear bag fibers receive group Ia sensory innervation, while nuclear chain fibers receive group II.

Golgi tendon organs are fascicles of collagen fibrils that receive myelinated group Ib sensory innervation. Attached to tendons on one end and 20 to 30 muscle fibers on the other, what function does this structure serve?

Golgi tendon organs are encapsulated sensory nerves that detect changes in muscle tension and respond to strong muscle contractions by inhibiting subsequent muscle contractions. Unlike muscle spindles, these collagen-based receptors have no contractile or motor function or innervation.

CARDIAC MUSCLE

Cardiac muscle cells are usually mono- or binucleate, branching cells with striations and intercalated disks. What are intercalated disks, and how do they function?

An intercalated disk is an intercellular protein plaque that contains three structures critical to cardiac myocyte function—desmosome, fascia adherents, and gap junction. Those structures mediate cell-cell adhesion, link and anchor structural fibers (actin) between neighboring cells, and electrically couple the cells into a **syncytium** for unified contraction, respectively.

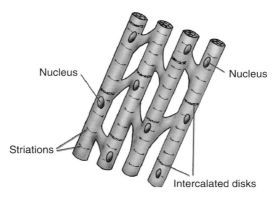

Figure 4.3   Cardiac muscle.

Cardiac myocytes differ ultrastructurally from skeletal muscle fibers in two subtle but functionally important ways—they contain lipid droplets rather than glycogen granules, and they have significantly more mitochondria and vascularization. What is the functional importance of these differences?

Sixty percent of cardiac myocyte metabolic energy is obtained from lipid stores, whereas skeletal muscle, especially type II fibers, use carbohydrate stores. Cardiac myocytes have greater metabolic demands than skeletal muscle, generating nearly all of their energy from aerobic processes; thus they have a greater need for mitochondria and arterial blood flow.

Where are T-tubules located in a cardiac myocyte?

T-tubules are located at the **Z-bands** in a dyad with small terminal cisternae.

How do the sarcomeres of cardiac myocytes in a blood-filled ventricle differ from those in an empty ventricle?

According to **Starling's law of the heart**, sarcomeres stretched by a blood-filled ventricle have a much greater force of contraction than those in an empty ventricle. That contractile force increases to a point and begins to decline when sarcomeres are overstretched.

Atrial cardiac myocytes contain abundant granules in a juxtanuclear region devoid of contractile proteins. What is the physiologic significance of those atrial granules?

Atrial granules contain the hormones **atrial** and **brain natriuretic factors (peptides)**, which act in the kidneys as sodium-wasting diuretics to reduce blood pressure.

Skeletal, cardiac, and smooth muscle cells all have Ca^{2+} channels in their cell membranes and SR within the cells. Despite those ultrastructural similarities, skeletal muscle is unaffected by Ca^{2+} channel blockade while cardiac and smooth muscle are potently blocked. What is the histologic basis for this pharmacologic difference?

Although all myocytes contain dihydropyridine Ca^{2+} channels, skeletal myocytes do not require Ca^{2+} entry through these channels to initiate a contraction. Instead, mechanical interactions between those channels and the SR release the intracellular Ca^{2+}, required for contraction.

Cardiac and smooth myocytes require extracellular Ca^{2+} to initiate a contraction due to Ca^{2+}-induced Ca^{2+} release from the SR.

SMOOTH MUSCLE

Smooth muscle comes in two forms— one type containing sheets of nonstriated, fusiform cells with tortuous nuclei and gap junctions, and a second type containing individual bundles of cells without gap junctions. What are those types of smooth muscle, and how do they function?

1. Visceral smooth muscle makes up the walls of hollow organs, like the intestine, uterus, and ureters.
2. Multiunit smooth muscle functions in fine, graded involuntary contractions of organs, like the iris.

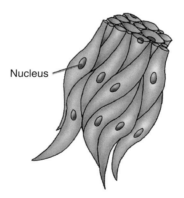

Figure 4.4 Smooth muscle.

What is the functional significance of gap junctions and unstable membrane potentials in visceral smooth muscle?

Gap junctions create a **syncytium** by electrically coupling smooth muscle cells. Since visceral smooth myocytes randomly depolarize, the addition of gap junctions makes **peristaltic contractions** possible.

Which skeletal muscle structures do smooth muscle dense bodies resemble?

Dense bodies resemble Z-bands; both function as anchors for actin filaments.

After Ca^{2+} flows into the smooth muscle cell, what protein binds Ca^{2+} to regulate contractions?

Calmodulin binds intracellular Ca^{2+} and drives the activation of myosin light chain kinase.

Besides Ca^{2+} concentration, what mechanism is important in regulating smooth muscle contraction?

Phosphorylation of the myosin heads by Ca^{2+}-calmodulin–activated myosin light chain kinase is critical for smooth muscle contraction. Phosphorylated myosin has increased myosin ATPase activity and increased binding affinity for actin.

Smooth muscle cells do not relax immediately after contraction. Rather they maintain their contracted state despite dephosphorylation of myosin and reduction in intracellular Ca^{2+} levels. By what mechanism does this occur, and how does it affect the energetics of the cell?

Though controversial, maintaining a constant contracted state appears to occur by a **latch-bridge mechanism** where myosin does not detach from the actin filaments. This process appears to occur with no energy expenditure by the smooth muscle cells.

CLINICAL CORRELATES AND VIGNETTES

A 26 yo M with no medical history passes out while running on a hot day after not drinking. In the ED his temperature is 105°F. His laboratory results show CK of 2000 IU/L, AST of 400 IU/L, and ALT of 66 IU/L. What is the diagnosis?

Heat stroke occurs when the body temperature is elevated for a prolonged period of time (> 105°F for > 15 minutes). This can cause multiple organ system damage, especially of the muscles. As the muscles break down, a rhabdomyolysis-like phenomenon emerges with extremely high CK levels.

A 52 yo homeless F with HIV has recurrent episodes of chest pain and hemoptysis over the course of a year. She has persistent night sweats and unintentional weight loss despite unchanged diet or exercise. Where is she losing weight from?

Homelessness and HIV infection are both risk factors for developing TB. Her pulmonary symptoms and nightly fevers are consistent with TB as well. In TB, as in some neoplasms, elevated levels of TNF-α can lead to muscle wasting, known as **cachexia**. Cachexia is separate from general wasting of fat and muscles, as is seen in starvation, or the muscle wasting of age, as is seen in sarcopenia.

A 14 yo M starts having difficulty climbing stairs and jumping. When he stands up, he frequently uses his hands to help push himself upright. He has developed enlarged calves, and his pediatrician is concerned over a possible new heart murmur. His mother reports that her father had a "muscle disease." What is the diagnosis?

A **muscular dystrophy**. This picture, in which the symptoms start later (teens) and there is cardiac involvement, is more common for **Becker muscular dystrophy** than Duchenne. Both types are caused by defects in dystrophin, encoded on the X chromosome. Dystrophin helps anchor muscle fibers to the extracellular matrix, preventing damage upon contraction.

CHAPTER 5

Nervous System

NERVOUS SYSTEM

Controller and supporter cells make up what two cell categories of nervous tissue?	Neurons and glial cells, respectively

EMBRYOLOGY

From what embryologic layer does neural tissue originate?	Embryonic ectoderm
From what embryonic structure does the central nervous system (CNS) and peripheral nervous system (PNS) develop?	The CNS originates from the neural tube and the PNS from flanking neural crest cells.
What are the three most common causes of congenital malformations of the CNS?	Note the mnemonic: **CSF** **C**losure—failure of the neural tube to close **S**eparation—failure of the neural tube to separate from the surface ectoderm **F**usion—failure of fusion of the vertebral arches
Prenatal diagnosis of neural tube defects (NTDs) is dependent on which marker?	High α-fetoprotein levels in maternal serum or amniotic fluid
Which nutrient is added to a variety of foods to prevent NTDs?	**Spina bifida** and **anencephaly**, the two most common forms of NTDs, occur in 1/1000 US pregnancies and in an estimated 300,000 newborns worldwide each year. Prenatal intake of **folic acid** is effective in preventing NTDs.

NEURONS

What are the main parts of a neuron?	Remember **ABCDs**: **a**xons, **b**outons, **c**ell body, **d**endrites, and **s**ynapses
What are the key histologic features of the cell body or perikaryon?	1. Prominent, central, pale staining **nucleus** 2. **Nissl bodies**—dense, basophilic free ribosomes, and rough endoplasmic reticulum 3. **Tapering axon hillock** containing abundant ion channels
In general, what does the size of the body of the neuron indicate about its function?	Cell body size correlates with the **axon length** and the **proximity of the effect**—large cells with long axons influence distant activities whereas small cells with short axons influence local activities.
How are axons different from dendrites?	Think, "**SAMBA**"—**S**ize, **A**rborization, **M**yelination, **B**idirectional transport, **A**xon hillock, and initial segment.
What type of synapse do gap junctions exemplify?	Electrical synapse
What other general feature of a neuron determines its function?	**Shape**—neurons come in four shapes: multipolar, bipolar, pseudounipolar, and unipolar. In general, multipolar cells are motor or efferent neurons, bipolar cells are special sensory signal transducers or interneurons, and pseudounipolar cells are sensory or afferent neurons.

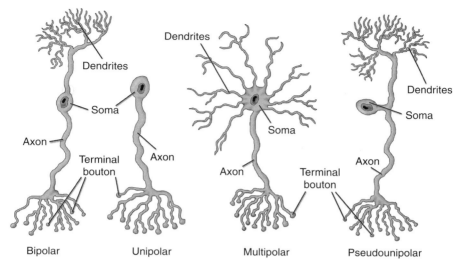

Figure 5.1   Neuron types.

GLIAL CELLS

Contrast oligodendrocytic myelination with Schwann cell–mediated myelination.	Oligodendrocytes myelinate multiple axons within CNS; Schwann cells myelinate a single axon within the PNS.
What are the histologic features of an oligodendrocyte?	These cells contain small, dark nuclei with a perinuclear halo (**fried egg appearance**) and extensive dendritic processes.

How do fibrous and protoplasmic astrocytes differ from each other?

See Table 5.1

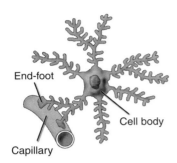

Figure 5.2   Protoplasmic astrocyte.

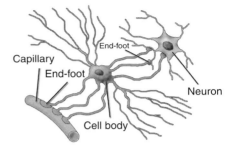

Figure 5.3   Fibrous astrocyte.

Table 5.1 Characteristics of Astrocytes

Type of Astrocyte	Location	Processes
Fibrous	White matter	Several, long processes
Protoplasmic	Gray matter	Abundant, short processes

Which neurotransmitters are typically metabolized by astrocytes?

Serotonin, γ-aminobutyric acid (GABA), and glutamate

Which extracellular ion concentration is modulated by astrocytes?

Potassium

What is the major function of an astrocyte?

To provide **support** for the interfaces between the pia and CNS and between the ependyma and CNS

What is a cellular marker for astrocytes?

The intermediate filament protein, glial fibrillary acidic protein (GFAP)

What histologic structure enables ependymal cells to filter and secrete cerebrospinal fluid (CSF)?

Cilia

What are the histologic features of an ependymal cell?

Ciliated, low columnar epithelial cells cast in folds or forming rosettes that line the brain ventricles

What other cell can be found among the ependymal cells?

Tanycytes. Elongated cells with long processes that connect the ventricles, brain parenchyma, and vasculature. These cells transport CSF to neurons in the hypothalamus.

Microglia are small, elongated cells with rod-shaped nuclei and bipolar dendritic processes. How do they differ from all other glial cells?

Belong to the mononuclear phagocytic system and **originate in the bone marrow**. All other glial cells originate from the neural tube.

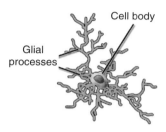

Cell body

Glial processes

Figure 5.4   Microglial cell.

Which cells are typically destroyed in multiple sclerosis?

Oligodendrocytes

An acoustic neuroma is an example of what type of tumor?

Schwannoma

What is gliosis?

Scarring in damaged areas of the brain; formed by astrocytes.

What percentage of intracranial tumors arise from glial cells?

Approximately 50%

CENTRAL NERVOUS SYSTEM

How does the nervous tissue of the cerebrum and cerebellum differ from that of the spinal cord?

Cerebral and **cerebellar cortices**: thin gray matter capsule with white matter core; islands of gray matter scattered throughout

Spinal cord: thick white matter capsule and an H-shaped gray matter core

How is the cerebral cortex organized?   Six layers:
I: molecular layer
II: external granular layer
III: external pyramidal layer
IV: internal granular layer
V: internal pyramidal layer
VI: fusiform layer

What are the histologic features of a Betz cell?   Giant, multipolar pyramidal cells with a large nucleus, prominent nucleolus, and abundant Nissl substance

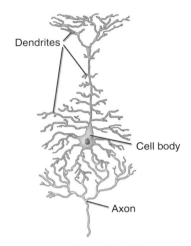

Figure 5.5   Pyramidal cell.

How is the cerebellar cortex organized?   Three layers: inner granular, middle Purkinje cell, and an outer molecular layer

Describe a cerebellar Purkinje cell.

Large multipolar cell with extensive arborizing dendrites; these cells function in maintaining balance and smoothing motor coordination.

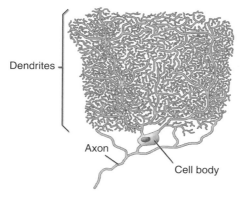

Figure 5.6 Cerebellar Purkinje cell.

Besides Lewy bodies, what other inclusion abnormalities are found in patients with Parkinson's disease?

Loss of neuromelanin from the substantia nigra and locus ceruleus

What intracytoplasmic inclusions are most commonly associated with Alzheimer's disease?

Hirano bodies, found in the hippocampus

MENINGES

How are the layers of the meninges ordered in the skull?

DAP—dura mater, arachnoid, pia

What is the function of the finger-like projections in the dura mater that contain CSF crystals?

Arachnoid villi facilitate the reabsorption of CSF into dural venous blood.

What are the two tightly apposed fibrous connective tissue layers of the dura?

1. **Outer periosteum**
2. **Inner meningeal** layer

What layer of the dura forms the four intracranial reflections?

1. Falx cerebri
2. Falx cerebelli
3. Tentorium cerebelli
4. Diaphragma sellae

What structures make up the blood-brain barrier (BBB)?

Vascular endothelial cells with tight junctions constitute the barrier function. They are induced and reinforced by astrocytic foot processes.

If pia mater invests the brain and blood vessels, why does it not constitute the BBB?

Pia mater is loose connective tissue lined by squamous cells. Junctions between pial squames are not tight enough to regulate the passage of materials between the blood and the parenchyma of the brain.

What is the choroid plexus?

A specialized fenestrated capillary tuft containing dense connective tissue that is invested by modified ependymal cells.

Why is a breech of the choroid plexus not considered a breech of the BBB?

Although continuous with the vasculature of the brain, the choroid plexus is not contained within the brain parenchyma. Thus it is not invested by the underlying astrocytes. Substances that breech the choroid plexus are actually contained within the ventricles, a space continuous with the subarachnoid space.

In what part of the CNS is the BBB absent?

The BBB does not exist in several spaces where direct access to the blood stream is critical:

1. The median eminence and posterior pituitary, where protein hormones are released
2. The chemoreceptor trigger zone or area postrema
3. The lamina terminalis and pineal gland

PERIPHERAL NERVOUS SYSTEM

How do unmyelinated neurons in the PNS differ from those in the CNS?

Unmyelinated peripheral axons are **ensheathed** by neighboring Schwann cells, the peripheral glia. However, unmyelinated central axons run naked and are not associated with any type of supportive oligodendrocyte.

How do unmyelinated and myelinated peripheral nerve fibers differ?

Myelinated fibers have **nodes of Ranvier** and undergo **saltatory conduction**; unmyelinated fibers do not have nodes of Ranvier.

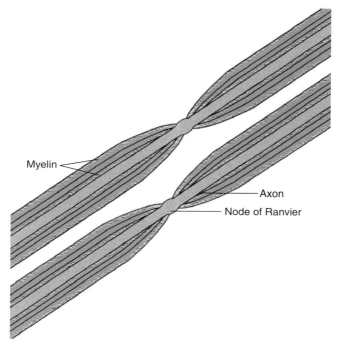

Myelin

Axon

Node of Ranvier

Figure 5.7   Myelinated axons.

How are peripheral nerves organized?

Epineurium (outer) surrounds the whole peripheral nerve.

Perineurium (middle) surrounds a bundle of axons.

Endoneurium (inner) surrounds individual axons.

What histologic feature of peripheral nerves approximates the function of the BBB?

Tight junctions of perineural epithelioid cells

During microsurgical reconnection of a transected nerve, which peripheral nerve layer must be reattached for the nerve to be functional?

Perineurium, which acts as a permeability barrier

Explain why peripheral neuropathy is sometimes seen in cancer patients who are treated with microtubule inhibitors, such as paclitaxel.	Microtubules are involved in axonal transport of neurotransmitters to the synapse. Inhibition of microtubule activity by chemotherapy will affect these neuronal processes.
What histologic feature of sensory ganglia makes it unique among the ganglia?	**Pseudounipolar neurons** are only located in sensory ganglia where there are **no synapses**.
What is the supportive (glial) cell of the sensory ganglion?	Satellite cells
What are the key differences between parasympathetic and sympathetic ganglia?	See Table 5.2

Table 5.2 Characteristics of Parasympathetic and Sympathetic Ganglia

Type of Ganglia	Location	Supporting cells
Parasympathetic	Target organs	Not encapsulated No supporting glial cells
Sympathetic	Sympathetic chain	Encapsulated Have supporting glial cells

CLINICAL CORRELATES AND VIGNETTES

Years following an ischemic stroke, a 66 yo M dies of a massive heart attack. During the autopsy, the infarcted region of his brain is examined to reveal what dominant cell type in his brain near the stroke region?

Astrocytes form scar tissue within the nervous tissue.

Following an episode of vision loss from optic neuritis 10 years ago, a 50 yo F was diagnosed with multiple sclerosis, an autoimmune-demyelinating disorder of the CNS. What would histologic examination of a biopsy of her optic nerve show?

The key is the timeline of the inflammatory response. Lesions early in the disease process show microglial proliferation and phagocytosis of degenerating myelin sheaths. Once the inflammation resolves, astrocytes replace microglia, surround the axon, and proliferate into a **gliotic scar**.

81 yo F p/w progressively declining physical and cognitive abilities. Over 3 years, her resting tremor has become b/l, her gait small and shuffling, and her balance poor. Seeing her for the first time, the rotating medical student quickly diagnoses her condition, but the student mistakenly treats it with dopamine. What is this condition, and what histologic structures contribute to the ineffectiveness of dopamine?

This patient has **Parkinson's disease**, which is treated with L-dopa, a dopamine precursor that accesses the brain via a large neutral amino acid transporter. Dopamine is not an effective therapy because, like all other neurotransmitters that circulate within the blood, it is unable to cross the BBB.

CHAPTER 6

Cardiovascular and Lymphatics

HEART

What three tissue layers are present in the heart?	1. Endocardium 2. Myocardium 3. Epicardium
What cell type makes up the endocardium?	A single layer of squamous endothelial cells
Is there a tissue layer between the endocardium and the myocardium?	Yes, there is a subendocardial layer, which is a network of loose connective tissue consisting of nerves, vessels, and branches of Purkinje cells.
Unlike the endocardium, the epicardium contains an abundance of what cell type?	Fat cells
What is the relationship between the epicardium and the pericardium?	The epicardium forms the visceral pericardium. The pericardium consists of two layers: the inner serosal layer (visceral pericardium) and the fibrous outer layer (parietal pericardium).
What separates the visceral from parietal pericardium?	The pericardial cavity contains a thin film of **pericardial fluid** that separates and decreases friction between the two layers.

What are two pathological conditions of the pericardium?

1. **Pericarditis** is inflammation of the pericardium manifesting as chest pain.
2. **Pericardial tamponade** results from an accumulation of fluids in the pericardial space.

What is Beck's triad?

The three clinical manifestations of pericardial tamponade are described as:

1. **Hypotension** due to decreased stroke volume
2. **Muffled heart sounds** due to pericardial fluid accumulation
3. **Elevated jugular venous pressure** due to impaired venous return to the heart

What are the three functions of the pericardium?

1. The pericardium **positions the heart** within the mediastinum.
2. It **prevents extreme dilation** of the heart during sharp rises in intracardiac volume.
3. It **limits the spread of infection** from the lungs.

Which is the thickest of the three layers of the heart?

Myocardium

What are the two major groups of cells in the myocardium?

1. Contractile cells
2. Impulse generating cells

How do cardiac myocytes differ from skeletal myocytes with regard to mitochondria?

Mitochondria compose 40% of the cell volume of cardiac muscle cells and only 2% of the cell volume of skeletal muscle cells, demonstrating the significance of aerobic metabolism for the heart.

If skeletal muscle cells attach to bones, to what structures do cardiac muscle cells attach?

Cardiac myocytes attach to the fibrous skeleton of the heart, which consists of dense collagenous connective tissue. The three components of this skeleton are the fibrous annuli, which support the atrioventricular and pulmonic valves, the fibrous trigone which supports the aortic valve, and the upper membranous portion of the interventricular septum.

What additional function does the fibrous skeleton serve in the heart?

The connective tissue skeleton also acts as an **insulator** between the atria and ventricles, ensuring that electrical conduction will occur along the designated routes.

How does cardiomyocyte contraction relate to the heart's capacity to pump blood?

The Frank-Starling mechanism describes the relationship between left ventricular end-diastolic volume (or pressure) and stroke volume. Briefly, increased venous return or preload stretches cardiac myocytes, which in turn stretches sarcomeres to optimize cross bridging. Better cross bridging results in greater contraction such that there is a greater stroke volume. Thus, the molecular basis for the Frank-Starling curve is an optimization of sarcomere cross bridging.

What is the difference between the sarcolemma and sarcoplasmic reticulum (SR)?

The sarcolemma is the cardiomyocyte surface membrane; the SR is separate and surrounds each myofibril. Note: A cardiomyocyte contains many myofibrils.

What ion stored in the SR is responsible for cardiac contraction?

Calcium. Inotropic drugs such as digoxin increase cardiac muscle contractility and thus cardiac output by increasing the concentration of Ca^{2+} in the cytoplasm. Digoxin inhibits the Na^+-K^+ ATPase on the basolateral membranes of cardiac cells, which in turn increases the intracellular concentration of Na^+. Through stimulation of Na^+-Ca^{2+} exchange, the intracellular concentration of Ca^{2+} is increased.

How are action potentials that propagate on the sarcolemma transmitted to the SR?

The T-tubule system is an extension of the sarcolemma that runs transversely through the cardiomyocyte. Action potentials are propagated along the T-tubule system and lead to Ca^{2+} release from the SR.

How are cardiac cells electrically and mechanically linked?

Intercalated disks electrically and mechanically link cardiomyocytes, which allow them to function as an integrated unit. Three specialized intercellular junctions occur within the intercalated disks: **gap junctions, fascia adherens junctions,** and **maculae adherens junctions (desmosomes).**

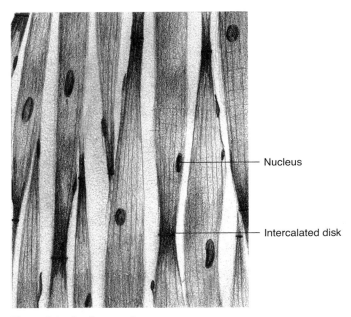

Nucleus

Intercalated disk

Figure 6.1   Cardiac muscle.

What is the function of the gap junctions?

They provide a low-resistance pathway across the membranes of adjoining cells that allows for the passage of ions and thus synchronous beating of cardiomyocytes.

What is the function of fascia adherens junctions?

They anchor actin filaments in each cell to the plasma membrane and provide a link between the plasma membranes of adjacent cells. They link the contractile filaments between cells to enable uniform contraction.

What is the function of desmosomes?

They provide adhesions between the plasma membranes of adjacent cells. They link to intermediate filaments, not actin.

Are atrial myocytes identical to ventricular myocytes?

No, ventricular myocytes, which contract against a higher resistance, are **larger** than atrial myocytes. Furthermore, atrial cells at baseline, unlike ventricular cells, contain **electron dense granules composed of atrial natriuretic factor** (ANF), a hormone released in response to atrial stretching. ANF functions to relax vascular smooth muscle and promote water and salt excretion by the kidneys. Note: Ventricular cardiomyocytes may express ANF when stressed in conditions such as congestive heart failure (CHF) and pulmonary hypertension.

Which cells are responsible for the initiation of a heartbeat? How?

The **cells of the sinoatrial (SA) node**, located near the entrance of the superior vena cava, initiate the heartbeat. These cells gradually depolarize during phase 4 of the action potential. This gradual depolarization allows the cells to spontaneously reach the threshold at which a new action potential is automatically triggered.

From the SA node, to which cells does the cardiac impulse propagate?

The cardiac impulse originates in the SA node and travels to the cells of the atrioventricular (AV) node, which is located in the right atrium. From the AV node, the impulse travels to the bundle of His.

What is the functional significance of the branching pattern of the cells of the bundle of His?

The bundle divides into one right and three left bundle branches that conduct the impulses via the Purkinje fibers to the ventricular cardiomyocytes.

ARTERIES, CAPILLARIES, AND VEINS

What are the three types of arteries?

1. Elastic (large)
2. Muscular (medium)
3. Arteriole (small)

What are their functions?

Elastic arteries—receive blood directly from the heart

Muscular arteries—deliver blood to organs

Arterioles—control blood pressure and distribution of blood to capillary beds

What are the major layers of the artery?

1. **Tunica intima**—internal endothelial layer
2. **Tunica media**—middle smooth muscle layer with elastin
3. **Tunica adventitia**—outside layer composed of fibroblasts and collagen fibers

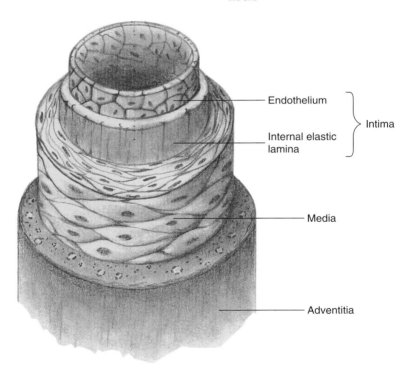

Figure 6.2   Artery layers.

Which layer is thickest and why?

Tunica media. It consists primarily of circumferentially arranged smooth muscle cells and regulates the diameter of the vessel.

Where are the internal and external elastic membranes?

The internal elastic membrane is found between the tunica intima and tunica media. The external elastic membrane is located between the media and adventitia in larger arteries.

What are vasa vasorum?

Vessels that feed the outer layers of veins and large arteries, areas that are not exposed to luminal nutrients. They are found in the tunica adventitia.

What type of collagen is found in vessels?

Type I—arteries
Type IV—basal lamina

Why do coronary arteries generally have a thicker tunica media than pulmonary arteries?

The thickness of the tunica media correlates with the blood pressure to which the vessel is exposed. Since coronary arteries are exposed to a higher blood pressure than the pulmonary circulatory vessels, the coronaries will have a thicker tunica media.

Where is blood pressure predominantly regulated?

At the level of the arteriole, blood pressure is determined by the amount of resistance found in these vessels, which is inversely related to vessel diameter. Thus an increase in arteriole diameter leads to a decrease in vessel resistance, and vice versa.

What are the major differences between veins and arteries?

Veins have **thinner walls**, especially the tunica media, and **thicker adventitia**. Medium-sized veins coursing through the limbs also have **valves**, which help distinguish them from arteries.

What are the blood pathways between arteries and veins?

Artery → arteriole → capillary → venule → vein

What are the three types of capillaries?   Based on the three types of capillary endothelium:

1. Continuous capillary
2. Fenestrated capillary
3. Sinusoidal/discontinuous capillary

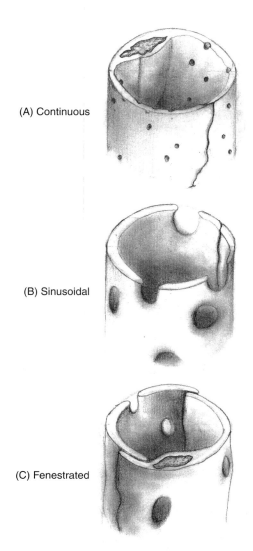

(A) Continuous

(B) Sinusoidal

(C) Fenestrated

Figure 6.3   Capillary types.

What are the differences between these three types of capillaries?

Continuous—no pores in the continuous endothelium; found in connective tissue, neural tissue, and exocrine glands

Fenestrated—some endothelial pores; found in tissues where rapid exchange between the blood and tissue is required (eg, kidneys, intestines, and endocrine glands)

Sinusoidal—large endothelial pores; found in the liver and hematopoietic organs (bone marrow and spleen)

What are the carotid sinuses and where are they located?

Located just above the bifurcation of the common carotid arteries. The carotid sinuses are highly innervated regions that constantly measure and regulate blood pressure.

What are the histologic characteristics of a carotid sinus?

The carotid sinus contains a thin media and an adventitia with specialized sensory nerve fibers.

How is blood vessel tone controlled by the nervous system?

The vasomotor center in the medulla oblongata controls the vasomotor tone of medium and small arteries by transmitting impulses through the spinal cord sympathetic ganglia.

What is reactive hyperemia, and how does it contribute to local vessel tone regulation?

Reactive hyperemia is the phenomenon whereby an organ experiences a transient increase in blood flow immediately following a brief period of ischemia (eg, removal of a tourniquet). During the period of occlusion, tissue hypoxia and an accumulation of vasomotor metabolites cause arteriole dilation. When flow is reestablished, the tissues are oxygenated and vasomotor metabolites flushed out allowing the vessel tone to return to normal.

What are carotid bodies?

Epithelioid cell chemoreceptors surrounded by numerous sinusoids embedded in the connective tissue of the adventitia at the bifurcation of the common carotids and the aortic arch.

What do carotid bodies sense?

O_2, CO_2, and pH via the vagus (CN X) and glossopharyngeal (CN IX) nerves

Where do angiotensin-converting enzyme inhibitors primarily act?

Lung capillary endothelium

What congenital diseases predispose someone to aortic dissection?

Turner syndrome and connective tissue disorders, including Marfan and Ehlers-Danlos syndromes.

What is the genetic defect in Ehlers-Danlos syndrome that predisposes one to aortic dissection and aortic aneurysm?

Defects in type III collagen formation

What is the etiology of aortic dissection in Marfan syndrome?

A *fibrillin* gene mutation leads to a weakening of the intimal layer and medial degeneration.

A third-year medical student is looking at the fundus of a patient's eye and sees two vessels traveling together, one significantly larger than the other. Which is the vein?

The vein is the larger vessel. In general, veins have a larger diameter than arteries and act more as capacitance vessels.

Coronary artery bypass grafting (CABG) is a common treatment for coronary artery stenosis. The graft sometimes uses the great saphenous vein from the leg to connect the aorta to the distal coronary artery. What venous feature must the cardiac surgeon consider when placing the graft in the heart?

The saphenous vein must be oriented opposite to its original orientation in the leg because veins contain semilunar valves that restrict backflow and allow unidirectional flow.

LYMPHATIC VESSELS

How do lymph vessels differ from blood vessels?

Lymph vessels, like blood vessels, begin as capillaries in the periphery, merging together to form larger vessels.

Larger lymph vessels, like veins, contain valves and thus conduct fluid in one direction.

Lymph capillaries differ from blood capillaries in that they are close-ended tubules that contain a single layer of endothelial cells, without fenestrations, basal laminae, or zonula occludentes.

In what parts of the body are lymphatic vessels not found?

Central nervous system, cartilage, teeth, and bone.

What is the path of lymph fluid flow?

Lymph capillaries → afferent lymph vessels → lymph node → efferent lymph vessels → lymph ducts → venous system

Where does the lymphatic system drain into the venous system?

The **thoracic duct** and the **right lymphatic duct,** which empty into the venous system. The thoracic duct collects lymph from almost the entire body (except the right upper quadrant) and drains into the systemic circulation at the junction of the left subclavian and left internal jugular veins. The right thoracic duct drains into the junction of the right subclavian and right internal jugular veins.

What part of the body does the right lymphatic duct drain?

It drains from the right arm, right upper trunk, right side of head and neck, and left lower lobe of the lungs. The rest of the body is drained by the thoracic duct.

LYMPH NODES

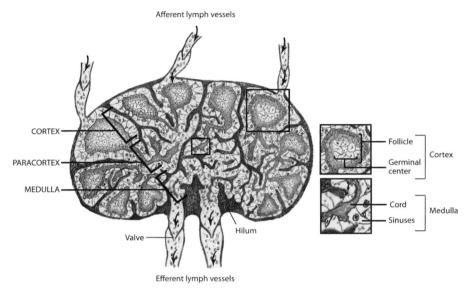

Figure 6.4   Lymph node.

What are the main compartments of a lymph node?	Cortex, paracortex, medulla (medullary cords and sinuses), sinuses
What is the pathway of lymphatic fluid through the lymph node?	Afferent lymphatic vessel → cortical sinus → medullary sinus → hilum → efferent lymphatic vessel
Where is the cortex located in the lymph node, and what cell types are present in the cortex?	It is situated on the **periphery of the lymph node** and contains mostly lymphocytes arranged in circular **follicles**.
What is the function of a follicle, and what cell types are found there?	It is the site where B-cells gather and proliferate. Memory and naive B-cells expand to form lymphoid nodules when exposed to foreign antigens. B-cells expressing surface IgM reside in the germinal center, while those expressing surface IgD reside in the mantle.

What is the histologic difference between primary and secondary follicles?

Secondary follicles are pale in the center because they have germinal centers.

Primary follicles are darker and do not have germinal centers.

Where is the paracortex (deep cortex), and what are the predominant cell types?

Paracortex: located between the cortex and medulla, lacking lymphoid follicles. This is where many T-cells move from blood to lymph. T-cells are sensitized to circulating antigens, proliferate, and are activated before being disseminated to peripheral sites.

What compartments make up the medulla of the lymph node?

Medullary sinuses and medullary cords

What is the function of medullary cords, and what cells are found there?

The medullary cords are extensions of lymphoid tissues from the paracortex into the medulla. Plasma cells mature and secrete antibodies. The cords contain B-lymphocytes, mainly plasma cells and macrophages.

What are medullary sinuses, and what cells are found there?

Medullary sinuses are lymph-filled dilated areas between medullary cords. Macrophages and lymphocytes are found in the sinuses, where they sample lymphatic contents flowing in from the periphery and function in antigen processing and presentation.

CLINICAL CORRELATES AND VIGNETTES

A 77 yo M with a h/o HTN, type 2 diabetes, and a 40-pack year smoking history comes to the ED with crushing substernal chest pain radiating to his left shoulder. His HR is 100 beats/min and BP is 100/50 mm Hg. His ECG shows ST elevations in I, aVL, and V_3 to V_6. His troponin I is elevated. Would you expect the ratio of this patient's tunica intima to tunica media to be higher or lower than a healthy 20-year-old man?

Higher. DM, smoking, and HTN are risk factors for forming atherosclerotic lesions, the cause of this patient's MI. Atherosclerotic vessels undergo intimal hyperplasia as lipids enter the intima via small nicks in the endothelium and are oxidized. Macrophages migrate into the vessel wall and engulf oxidized LDLs, leading to intimal thickening or a fatty streak. As the layer thickens, smooth myocytes enter the intima and secrete connective tissue changing the fatty streak into the more dangerous "fibrous plaque," which can rupture and cause complete occlusion of a coronary artery.

A 45 yo M presents to the ED with CP, SOB, and a cold sweat. He is noticeably irritated and uncomfortable, moving about profusely to ease his pain. An ECG done on the scene does not demonstrate an abnormal Q wave. However, the patient does have laboratory evidence of an infarct. Where is the location of the infarct, and what is the function of this location?

Prolonged **subendocardial ischemia** results in a non–Q-wave infarction. ECG abnormalities that appear with this condition include the following: a prolonged QT interval, an increased T wave, a flipped T wave, and a depressed ST segment. Located between the endocardium and the myocardium, the subendocardium houses the cells of the cardiac conduction system (Purkinje fiber cells), which function in transmitting impulses throughout the ventricular myocardium. Like watershed areas, this location is particularly susceptible to ischemia because of its limited perfusion during systole (due to myocardial contraction) and diastole (due to high intraventricular pressures).

A 65 yo M with a h/o HTN comes to the ED with a tearing and ripping pain in his chest that radiates to his back. Which parts of the aortic wall have separated?

Aortic dissection occurs when there is an intimal laceration allowing blood to enter the vessel wall. The blood most often travels along the tunica media dissecting between the middle to outer third of that layer.

A 25 yo F comes to the ED with a HR of 135 beats/min feeling light-headed and dizzy. Her ECG shows a narrow complex tachycardia with no P waves. She is diagnosed with AV nodal reentry tachycardia. The attending starts rubbing her neck, and her heart returns to normal rate and sinus rhythm. What happened?

Carotid sinus massage increases parasympathetic outflow to the heart and slows conduction through the AV node, allowing the heart to resume a normal rate and rhythm.

CHAPTER 7

Respiratory System

UPPER RESPIRATORY TRACT

What are the anatomical spaces of the upper respiratory tract? How do they affect air as it is inspired?

1. Nasal cavity
2. Paranasal sinuses
3. Nasopharynx

The upper respiratory tract serves to warm, filter, and humidify air as it is inspired. Paranasal sinuses are chambers for speech resonance.

What kind of epithelium lines the upper respiratory tract?

Pseudostratified columnar epithelium

What are the main cell types present in pseudostratified respiratory epithelium?

1. Ciliated columnar cells
2. Mucus secreting goblet cells
3. Brush cells with microvilli
4. Basal cells

Which cells function primarily to condition inspired air?

Ciliated columnar cells and goblet cells

What cell type acts as the sensory receptors for basal free nerve endings?

Brush cells

What special feature of pseudostratified columnar epithelial cells aids in mucus clearance?

The cilia present on the pseudostratified epithelium of the large airways work in coordination to propel mucus and particles toward the larynx, where it is swallowed. This phenomenon is called the **mucociliary elevator**.

What mucus-secreting cells are found in abundance in the upper respiratory tract?

Goblet cells as well as mucus glands secrete a thin layer of mucus that serves to trap foreign particles.

What are the major histologic features of the vestibule of the nasal cavity?

1. Transition from keratinized stratified squamous to pseudostratified ciliated columnar epithelium
2. Terminal hair follicles
3. Sebaceous and sweat glands

What are swell bodies, and what are their functions in the nasal vestibule?

Swell bodies are **large venous plexuses** in the conchae. They swell to divert air through the opposite nasal fossa, allowing the mucosa to recover from dehydration.

What types of muscles are the intrinsic and extrinsic laryngeal muscles?

Striated skeletal muscle

What cellular characteristics are present to reduce infection in respiratory epithelium but not in stratified squamous epithelium?

Stratified squamous epithelium contains **no cilia**; thus, it is more vulnerable to colonization and infection than respiratory epithelium.

LOWER RESPIRATORY TRACT

What are the anatomic divisions of the lower respiratory tract?

1. Larynx
2. Trachea
3. Bronchi
4. Bronchioles
5. Alveoli

What are the contents of the larynx, and what are their functions?

The larynx contains both true and false vocal cords, which protect the trachea against foreign bodies and create sound.

What structures are contained in the larynx that are essential for phonation?

Both the true and false vocal cords are contained in the larynx. Each "true" vocal cord contains a striated vocalis muscle.

What kind of cartilage is found in the trachea? What is its function?

C-shaped hyaline cartilage rings allow expansion and recoil of the trachea during respiration and prevent collapse.

Despite their common embryologic origins, how does the trachea differ histologically from the esophagus?

Unlike the esophagus that is lined by a stratified squamous epithelium, the trachea has respiratory epithelium and C-shaped hyaline cartilage, which keeps the tracheal lumen open. Smooth muscle links the open ends of the C-shaped rings, completing the circle and regulates the width of the lumen.

What are two prominent mucosal differences between the trachea and bronchi?

1. Bronchi contain complete rings, plates of hyaline cartilage, and subepithelial smooth muscle.
2. The trachea contains C-shaped cartilaginous rings, the ends of which are connected by smooth muscle strands.

What is the progress of airways down the respiratory tree from trachea to alveoli?

Trachea → primary (main) bronchi → secondary (lobar) bronchi → tertiary (segmental) bronchi → bronchioles → terminal bronchioles → respiratory bronchioles → alveolar ducts → alveolar sacs → alveoli

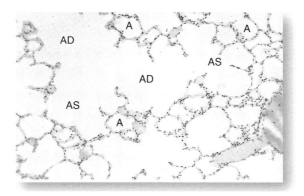

Figure 7.1 Alveolar sacs and ducts. AD, alveolar ducts; AS, alveolar sacs; A, alveoli. (*Reproduced, with permission, from Mescher AL.* Junqueira's Basic Histology: Text and Atlas. *12th ed. New York, NY: McGraw-Hill; 2009.*)

Simplification of the bronchiolar epithelium involves what histologic changes?	1. Change from pseudostratified to simple columnar epithelium 2. Reduction in number of goblet cells 3. Disappearance of cartilage
What is the histologic difference between a bronchus and bronchiole?	A bronchus has cartilage in its walls; bronchioles do not.
What structures lying within the lamina propria of bronchial branch points protect against wayward airborne microbes?	Secondary lymphoid follicles comprising the bronchus-associated lymphoid tissue (BALT)
How does the lamina propria change down the respiratory tree?	From the trachea to the bronchi, the lamina propria becomes denser with an increasing amount of elastin. In smaller airways, the lamina propria is separated from the submucosa by a discontinuous layer of smooth muscle.
How are Clara cells differentiated from other epithelial cells in the terminal bronchioles? What is their secretory product?	Clara cells are non-ciliated cells containing microvilli and apical secretory granules. They are the epithelial progenitor cells of the small airways (bronchioles) and therefore, important in repair. Clara cells produce a protein that is a component of surfactant.
Alveolar ducts differ from respiratory bronchioles in what way?	Density of alveoli—ducts contain more alveoli than bronchioles.
What is the distinctive structure of the type I pneumocyte (alveolar cell)?	Type I pneumocyte organelles are sequestered and their cytoplasm is attenuated to provide the thinnest layer possible for gas exchange.
How do types I and II alveolar cells differ from each other?	Remember, "**MS-NBC**" **M**icrovilli—type II cells have them, whereas type I cells do not. **S**hape—type II cells are cuboidal, whereas type I cells are squamous. **N**umber—type II cells are 33 times less numerous than type I cells. **B**odies—type II cells have lamellar and vesicular bodies, whereas type I cells do not. **C**ytoplasm—type I cells have sequestered organelles and attenuated cytoplasm.

What histologic layers make up the blood-air barrier in the lungs?

1. Type I alveolar cell membrane
2. Fused endothelial and epithelial basal laminae
3. Capillary endothelial cell membrane

What structures allow communication between the air spaces within clusters of neighboring alveoli?

Alveolar pores (pores of Kohn) function primarily as conduits for interalveolar movement of alveolar liquid, surfactant components, and macrophages and may provide collateral ventilation during atelectasis or obstruction.

What are the two main blood supplies to the lungs?

The pulmonary system supplies deoxygenated blood from the right side of the heart. The bronchial system provides oxygenated blood from the systemic circulation to the lower respiratory tract.

How many sets of arteries and veins are found in a bronchovascular bundle?

Two sets of arteries (pulmonary and bronchial) feed one set of veins (pulmonary).

PLEURA

How are visceral and parietal pleura similar?

Both contain mesothelia and underlying connective tissue layers composed of collagen and elastic fibers.

How are the visceral and parietal pleura different?

Visceral mesothelial cells form a continuous layer, whereas parietal mesothelial cells are discontinuous. The visceral connective tissue layer is thicker than the parietal connective tissue layer.

What is the significance of a discontinuous parietal pleural mesothelium?

The discontinuities are openings into the lymphatic drainage system.

What is the significance of a thinner parietal pleural connective tissue layer?

Facilitates transmembrane diffusion.

CLINICAL CORRELATES AND VIGNETTES

A 3 yo boy presents to the pediatrician with his mother who reports cough and frequent upper respiratory infections. She explains that this is his first time seeing a physician since he was born. On exam, you do not hear a heart beat upon auscultation of the left side of his chest. What histologic defect is the cause of this boy's infections?

This boy is suffering from **Kartagener's syndrome**, a congenital disorder also known as primary ciliary dyskinesia (PCD). PCD causes **defective ciliary movement and mucus clearance**, resulting in frequent upper and lower respiratory tract infections. During embryonic development, normal ciliary movement is responsible for organ placement; however, those with PCD develop situs inversus, a condition in which the major organs are reversed on the saggital plane from their normal positions in the body. This includes the heart, which in these patients is found on the right side of the chest.

A 34 yo F p/w a long h/o wheezing and SOB. She has no smoking history. On spirometry, severe airflow obstruction is seen. She has a forced expiratory volume in 1 second (FEV_1) that is only 30% of the predicted value. PE also reveals sublingual and scleral icterus and spider angiomata. Breath sounds are diminished throughout all lung fields. What underlying disease most likely accounts for this presentation? What trademark finding would be seen on lung biopsy?

α_1-**Antitrypsin (A1AT) deficiency** is a congenital disorder that primarily affects the liver and lungs. It increases the risk for COPD. The absence of A1AT enzyme disinhibits the activity of neutrophil elastase in the lungs causing alveolar destruction, eventually leading to emphysema. In the liver, abnormal A1AT proteins accumulate in hepatocytes leading to cirrhosis. Severe deficiency can lead to panacinar emphysema as early as age 30 years without a history of smoking.

A 12 yo girl complains of episodes of SOB, chest tightness, and wheezing after running with the cross-country team. You suspect an asthma exacerbation. What histologic abnormalities would you predict could be found in her bronchioles?

1. Smooth muscle thickening
2. Chronic inflammatory material surrounding the bronchioles (ie, lymphocytes)
3. Abundant mucus in the lumen
4. Decreased lumen diameter

CHAPTER 8

Endocrine

GENERAL

What is the fundamental difference between endocrine and exocrine glands? How does this difference occur developmentally?

The presence of **ducts**—endocrine ducts degenerate while exocrine ducts persist during development.

What are the two histologic arrangements of endocrine glands?

1. **Cords**—cell clumps located alongside dilated capillaries (eg, adrenal cortex)
2. **Follicles**—cell balls with a central core of noncellular material (eg, thyroid gland)

Using the histologic definition, what renal apparatus functions as an endocrine gland?

The **juxtaglomerular apparatus is a renin secreting** ductless cord of cells lying alongside the glomerulus. Secretion is stimulated by sympathetic activity and catecholamines and is inhibited by increased Na^+ and Cl^- reabsorption across the macula densa or increased afferent arterial pressure.

How do cardiomyocytes in the right atrium function as an endocrine gland?

Atrial muscle cells secrete **atrial natriuretic peptide (ANP)** in response to increased central venous pressure and stretch of atrial cardiac myocytes. ANP increases Na^+ excretion, decreases intravascular volume, and causes potent vascular dilation. Brain natriuretic peptide (BNP), a close relative of ANP, is monitored in cardiac disease as a marker of heart failure.

PITUITARY GLAND (HYOPHYSIS)

The pituitary is a trilobed bulb hanging from the hypothalamus by a stalk and sitting in the sella turcica of the sphenoid bone. What unique histologic feature of the stalk renders it susceptible to compromise in malignancy?

No meningeal covering; rather its stalk contains double layers of pia and arachnoid mater because the leptomeninges reflects back onto itself.

Development of a meningioma at this fold crushes the stalk leading to pituitary failure and hyperprolactinemia.

Pituicytes are the dominant nonendocrine cell type found in the posterior pituitary. However, two important hormones, antidiuretic hormone (ADH) and oxytocin, are found in abundance in this region. Explain this apparent contradiction.

Pituicytes are supportive astrocyte-like glial cells for the magnocellular neurons of the supraoptic and paraventricular nuclei. Those magnocellular neurons store hormones, ADH and oxytocin, in secretory granules in the dilated ends of the axons (Herring bodies) found in the posterior pituitary. The hormones in those axons are released into the posterior pituitary capillaries.

What is the function of the hormones released from Herring bodies in the posterior pituitary?

Vasopressin/ADH acts on the collecting ducts of the kidneys to increase water reabsorption and concentrate the urine.

Oxytocin stimulates uterine muscle contractions during labor, and it mediates the milk letdown reflex by stimulating myoepithelial cell contractions around the mammary lobules in the breast.

What is the general classification of cell types in the anterior pituitary?

Chromophils (acidophils and basophils) and chromophobes. Chromophobes are chromophils depleted of their secretory product at the time of fixation.

What are the five endocrine cell types found in the anterior pituitary, and how do they function?

See Table 8.1

Table 8.1 Endocrine Cells of the Anterior Pituitary And Their Functions

Endocrine Cells (Appearance)	Hormone	Function
Corticotrope (basophilic)	Adrenocorticotropic hormone (ACTH)	Stimulates adrenal cortex (zona fasciculata and reticularis) to secrete cortisol
Gonadotrope (basophilic)	Follicle-stimulating hormone (FSH)	Promotes ovarian follicle maturation from secondary to graafian follicles Stimulates spermatogenesis and Sertoli cell synthesis of androgen-binding protein
	Luteinizing hormone (LH)	Promotes ovulation, corpus luteum formation, and progesterone secretion in females Stimulates testosterone secretion from Leydig cells in males
Lactotrope (acidophilic)	Prolactin (PRL)	Promotes mammary gland growth, milk secretion, and maternal behavior
Somatotrope (acidophilic)	Growth hormone (GH)	Promotes skeletal growth, bone remodeling, and insulin-like growth factor (IGF)-1 secretion
Thyrotrope (basophilic)	Thyroid-stimulating hormone (TSH)	Stimulates thyroid gland growth and secretion of T_3 and T_4 (thyroxine)

How would a pathologist distinguish the type of anterior pituitary tumor?

Immunocytochemistry with antibodies to specific hormones is used to determine tumor origin and secretion.

Why does separating the anterior pituitary from the hypothalamus by severing the stalk lead to hyperprolactinemia and suppression of all other anterior pituitary hormones?

The hypothalamus synthesizes releasing and inhibitory factors (hormones), which stimulate hormone release from all anterior pituitary endocrine cells, except the lactotropes. For the lactotropes, the hypothalamus secretes dopamine, an inhibitor of prolactin release. Severing the pituitary stalk releases lactotropes from dopaminergic inhibition.

Pregnancy causes both the maternal and fetal pituitary glands to double in volume due to lactotrope hypertrophy and hyperplasia. What does this response to pregnancy reveal about lactotrope stimulation?

During pregnancy high levels of circulating estrogen stimulate lactotrope growth and division, causing the pituitary to double in volume. Because of the pituitary enlargement during pregnancy, it is vulnerable to ischemia especially if there has been severe hemorrhaging or hypotension peri- or postpartum. This can lead to hypopituitarism and is known as **Sheehan syndrome** or **postpartum pituitary necrosis**.

Prior to puberty, what anterior pituitary cell type has minimal development and activity?

Except in some cases of precocious puberty, gonadotropes are inactive from the neonatal period to the onset of puberty. In the absence of pulsatile gonadotropin-releasing hormone (GnRH) stimulation from the hypothalamus, the gonadotropes do not grow or release luteinizing hormone (LH) or follicle-stimulating hormone (FSH).

What effect does prolonged administration of glucocorticoids for anti-inflammatory purposes have on the pituitary gland? Why is high-dose glucocorticoid treatment tapered off rather than ended precipitously?

Long-term administration of glucocorticoids directly inhibits hypothalamic corticotropin-releasing hormone (CRH) and adrenocorticotropic hormone (ACTH) secretions. In the absence of stimulation, corticotropes and specific zones in the adrenal cortex atrophy. Abrupt termination of glucocorticoid therapy may precipitate an acute adrenal insufficiency syndrome and death.

ADRENAL GLAND

The adult adrenal gland contains a collagenous capsule surrounding four layers of cell cords positioned alongside capillaries. What are the different functional layers in the adult adrenal gland?

Outer cortex and **inner medulla**. The cortex subdivides into an aldosterone-producing zona glomerulosa, a cortisol-producing zona fasciculata, and an androgen-producing zona reticularis. The medulla comprises 30% of the adrenal mass and produces epinephrine and norepinephrine.

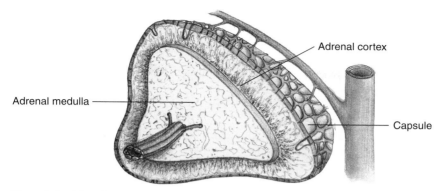

Figure 8.1   Adrenal gland.

What is the major functional difference between the fetal and adult adrenal glands?

The fetal adrenal cortex contains a large layer that produces sulfated androgens (dehydroepiandrosterone sulfate [DHEAS] and 16-hydroxy-DHEAS) that are converted to estrogens (estradiol and estriol, respectively) by the placenta. These estrogens prepare the uterine muscle for labor, and after birth, the fetal adrenal cortex rapidly involutes. During fetal life, the adrenal glands are larger than the kidneys because of the presence of the fetal adrenal cortex.

In the short term, why does pituitary failure lead to atrophy of the zona fasciculata and reticularis but no changes in the zona glomerulosa?

ACTH from the anterior pituitary stimulates and maintains cells in the zona fasciculata and reticularis. In contrast, angiotensin II, not ACTH, stimulates and maintains the zona glomerulosa in the short term. Long-standing hypopituitarism leads to atrophy of all three cortical zones, despite circulating levels of renin and angiotensin II.

Adrenal cortical cells are acidophilic with prominent lipid vacuoles and abundant smooth endoplasmic reticulum (SER) closely associated with mitochondria. What do those ultrastructural features indicate about the function of those cells?

These ultrastructural features are common to all steroid-secreting cells. Steroid biosynthesis occurs either de novo using acetate or by modifying dietary cholesterol through a series of compartmentalized reactions occurring in mitochondria and SER.

What are the critical enzymes associated with each region of the adrenal cortex, and what hormones do these regions produce?

See Table 8.2

Table 8.2 Adrenal Cortex Zones and the Secreted Enzymes and Hormones

Zone	Enzyme	Hormone
Zona glomerulosa	Aldosterone synthetase	Mineralocorticoids (aldosterone)
Zona fasciculata	11β-hydroxylase, 21-hydroxylase, 17α-hydroxylase	Glucocorticoids (cortisol and corticosterone)
Zona reticularis	11β-hydroxylase, 17α-hydroxylase, 17, 20 lyase	Androgens (DHEA, androstenedione, 11β-hydroxyandrostenedione)

The adrenals contain two distinct endocrine glands (cortex and medulla) with different embryologic origins (intermediate mesoderm and neural crest, respectively). Cortical function is stimulated hormonally either by ACTH or angiotensin II. How is medullary function stimulated?

The adrenal medulla is a sympathetic ganglion that receives **stimulatory, preganglionic** and **sympathetic innervation**. Medullary cell degranulation is a Ca^{2+}-dependent process occurring after synaptic ACh triggers Ca^{2+} entry through transmembrane cation channels.

Two cell types are found in the adrenal medulla based on the size of their cytoplasmic granules. The major cell type makes up 90% of the cells and contains large dense granules. The remaining minor type contains fewer and smaller, dense granules. What is the functional significance of this histologic observation?

Major cell type: contains phenylethanolamine N-methyltransferase (PNMT), the cortisol-induced enzyme required for epinephrine synthesis

Minor cell type: only contains norepinephrine, the catecholamine precursor to epinephrine

PANCREAS

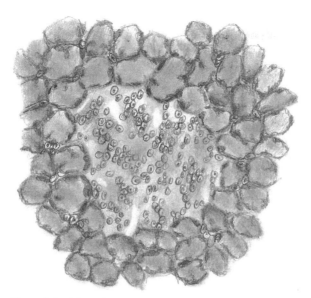

Figure 8.2   Islets of Langerhans in parenchyma.

Pancreatic islets of Langerhans cells form the endocrine part of the pancreas and comprise only 2% of the volume of the gland. What types of cells are found in the pancreatic islets, and what are their corresponding functions?

See Table 8.3

Table 8.3 Pancreatic Islet Cells and Function

Islet Cells (Histologic Appearance)	Hormone Produced	Function
α (peripheral location)	Glucagon	Elevates blood glucose, free fatty acid, and ketone levels
β (central location)	Insulin	Lowers blood glucose, free fatty acid, and ketone levels
δ (peripheral location)	Somatostatin	Inhibits islet cell secretions, gastric acid and CCK release, and slows gastric emptying
F (peripheral location)	Pancreatic polypeptide	Slows nutrient absorption

β cells in the islets are stimulated to release insulin via the following pathway: ATP inhibits K^+ channels, thus depolarizing the cell by reducing K^+ efflux; Ca^{2+} enters the cell mediating cytoplasmic vesicle fusion with the cell membrane, and insulin is released. How do glucose, glyburide, and catecholamines affect insulin release?

- **Glucose** generates ATP and increases insulin release.
- **Glyburide** (sulfonylurea) works directly on the K^+ channel, stimulating insulin release.
- **Catecholamines** inhibit insulin secretion via α_2-adrenergic stimulation. Although catecholamines also stimulate insulin via β-adrenergic activation, usually inhibition dominates, except in the presence of exogenous α-blockers or β-agonists.

THYROID GLAND

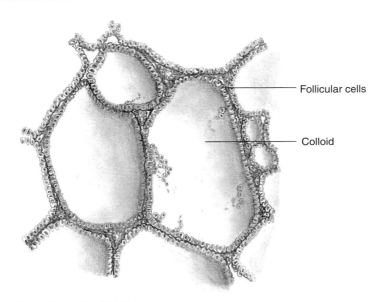

Figure 8.3   Thyroid follicles.

The thyroid gland differs from other endocrine organs. It is composed of spherical follicles, rather than cell cords. Describe the histologic organization of a thyroid follicle.

Spherical thyroid follicles contain a single epithelial cell layer surrounding a core of thyroglobulin-rich colloid composed of triiodothyronine (T_3) and thyroxine (T_4) residues.

The size of both the epithelial cell layer and the luminal colloidal sphere of a thyroid follicle varies based on its degree of stimulation and activity. Describe this variability and its corresponding hormonal state.

Inactive follicles under low thyroid-stimulating hormone (TSH) stimulation contain abundant colloid surrounded by a squamous epithelium. Follicles that actively elaborate T_3 and T_4 under high TSH stimulation contain minimal colloid surrounded by a high columnar epithelium. A cuboidal follicular epithelium appears in follicles that actively store luminal colloid.

Columnar follicular cells ingest colloid and hydrolyze its peptide bonds to release the prohormone T_4 and the effector hormone T_3 into the blood stream to act on target cells. How do target cells convert the prohormone T_4 into the more effective T_3?

Target cells contain the enzyme, 5'-deiodinase, which removes an iodine atom from T_4 to produce T_3. In order to function, this enzyme contains the rare amino acid, selenocysteine.

Hypothalamic thyrotropin-releasing hormone (TRH) stimulates cells in the anterior pituitary to secrete TSH, which in turn stimulates the thyroid gland to release T_4 and T_3. By negative feedback, T_4 and T_3 inhibit both TRH and TSH release. What histologic effect results from failure of this negative feedback mechanism?

Failure of the negative feedback mechanism causes prolonged stimulation of the thyroid gland by TSH leading to glandular enlargement, or a **goiter**.

Thyroid follicular cells are polarized and contain Na^+/I^- symporters (NIS) on their basal surfaces facing the capillaries and Na^+/K^+-ATPases on apical microvilli facing the colloid. How does this membrane polarity affect follicular cell function?

In a secondary active process maintained by Na^+/K^+-ATPase activity, iodide (I^-) is transported via NIS against its electrochemical gradient into the follicular cell. There I^- is oxidized to iodine by thyroid peroxidase and subsequently incorporated into thyroglobulin. This process is called **organification**.

Thyroid follicles contain two types of cells—follicular cells with microvilli and C (clear) cells also known as parafollicular cells without microvilli. How do these cells differ from each other functionally?

Follicular cells contain thyroglobulin, which deposits macromolecular thyroid hormone in luminal colloid and functions in cellular metabolism.

Parafollicular (clear) cells contain calcitonin, which lowers serum Ca^{2+} and phosphate levels by inhibiting osteoclast activity and increasing Ca^{2+} loss in the urine.

Remember the **two "C's"**: **C**lear cells and **C**alcitonin.

PARATHYROID GLAND

Parathyroid glands are four fatty, vascular structures embedded in the posterior capsule of the thyroid gland at the posterosuperior and inferior poles. What are the two major cell types found in these glands and how do they function?

1. Parathyroid hormone (PTH) from **chief cells** raises plasma Ca^{2+} levels by decreasing phosphate resorption in the proximal tubules, while increasing bone resorption and calcitriol formation in the kidneys.
2. **Oxyphil cell** function remains unknown, but the cells contain numerous mitochondria and produce PTH.

Histologically, resting chief cells can be differentiated from active cells based on the presence or absence, respectively, of cytoplasmic lipid droplets. How is PTH synthesis and release regulated in chief cells?

In states of low serum Ca^{2+}, PTH is constantly released from chief cells. However, when Ca^{2+} levels rise, Ca^{2+} activates the G-protein–coupled receptor in the cell membrane and initiates a phosphatidylinositol-mediated inhibition of PTH secretion.

Both primary and secondary hyperparathyroidism histologically reveal glandular hyperplasia, although they have different etiologies. Name some etiologies for primary and secondary hyperparathyroidism, and how one may distinguish between the two diseases.

Primary hyperparathyroidism is often caused by tumors, resulting in glandular hyperfunction and does not respond to negative feedback by Ca^{2+} levels. Both serum Ca^{2+} and PTH levels are high.

Secondary hyperparathyroidism, often caused by renal failure or Ca^{2+} malabsorption, results in low serum Ca^{2+} triggering normal functioning parathyroids to overproduce PTH.

In familial benign hypercalciuric hypocalcemia (FBHH), patients have higher than normal urinary Ca^{2+} and lower than normal serum Ca^{2+}. However, in familial hypocalciuric hypercalcemia (FHH), patients have the opposite—lower than normal urinary Ca^{2+} and higher than normal serum Ca^{2+}. How could disorders of the chief cell membrane Ca^{2+} receptor cause these two contrasting conditions?

Changes in the responsiveness of the Ca^{2+}-sensing receptor to serum calcium lead to inhibition of PTH release at abnormal serum Ca^{2+} levels. In FBHH, Ca^{2+} receptor mutations sensitize the receptor to lower serum Ca^{2+} causing inhibition of PTH release at lower serum Ca^{2+} concentrations. However, in FHH, Ca^{2+} receptor mutations desensitize the receptor to Ca^{2+} causing it to activate at higher than normal serum Ca^{2+} levels.

CLINICAL CORRELATES AND VIGNETTES

A 50 yo F p/w episodic H/A, sweating, and palpitations. She reports frequent onsets of dizziness when she stands, but never when she is sitting down or supine. These dizzy spells are associated with diaphoresis, weakness in the legs, and palpitations. An MRI and an MRA of the head and neck are unremarkable. Cardiac monitoring shows sinus tachycardia. Serum metabolites of epinephrine, norepinephrine, and dopamine are high. What would be found in the urine? What is her diagnosis?

> **Pheochromocytoma** results in high urine levels of catecholamine metabolites, such as metanephrines and normetanephrines. This is a neoplasm of the chromaffin cells arising from the adrenal glands.
>
> Remember the **Rule of 10's**.
>
> 10% malignant.
>
> 10% bilateral.
>
> 10% extra-adrenal.
>
> 10% calcify.
>
> 10% are in the pediatric population.
>
> 10% are familial.

A 51 yo M p/w H/A, erectile dysfunction, and reports decreased libido. On exam, his testicles are small b/l. On MRI, a sellar mass below the optic chiasm is evident. What would you expect to find elevated in his serum? What is his diagnosis?

> This patient has a **prolactinoma** and would have elevated levels of **prolactin.** This is the most common type of secretory pituitary tumor. Serum levels of prolactin are usually proportional to the size of the tumor mass.

A 40 yo F p/w palpitations, weight loss despite good appetite, irritability, and loose stools. She appears anxious. On exam, her HR is 120 beats/min but normotensive. She exhibits proptosis. Her thyroid glands are diffusely enlarged, and a thyroid bruit is audible. A radioiodine scan reveals increased uptake in the thyroid glands and increased blood flow is detected by Doppler ultrasonography. She is diagnosed with Graves disease. Describe the microscopic appearance of her thyroid gland.

> Follicular epithelial cells will increase in both number and size; scant colloid; small and closely packed follicles. Most patients have **TSH-R stimulating antibody** directed against the TSH receptor in the thyroid follicular epithelial membrane.

CHAPTER 9

Skin and Glands

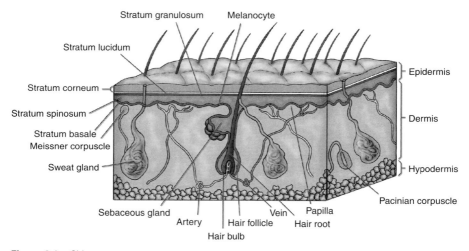

Stratum granulosum   Melanocyte
Stratum lucidum
Stratum corneum
Stratum spinosum
Stratum basale
Meissner corpuscle
Sweat gland
Epidermis
Dermis
Hypodermis
Pacinian corpuscle
Sebaceous gland   Vein   Papilla
Artery   Hair follicle   Hair root
Hair bulb

Figure 9.1   Skin.

ORGANIZATION

What are the three layers of the skin?

1. Epidermis
2. Dermis
3. Hypodermis

Which layer of the skin has the most diverse tissue and cellular composition?

Dermis

EPIDERMIS

What cell types are found in the epidermis?

Keratinocytes, melanocytes, Langerhans cells, and Merkel cells

Name the layers or strata of the epidermis in thick skin.

Stratum basalis, s. spinosum, s. granulosum, s. lucidum, and s. corneum

Melanocytes are round, pale staining, granular cells with dendritic extensions. What do the granules contain, and how do these cells function?

Eumelanin and **pheomelanin**. These granules are transferred to basal and spinous keratinocytes, where they surround the nucleus shielding it from ultraviolet (UV) radiation.

Skin color correlates with what histologic observation?

Number of melanin granules per keratinocyte

From which cell line are Langerhans cells derived?

Bone marrow–derived monocytes

Describe the histologic characteristics of Merkel cells.

Merkel cells contain **prominent cytoplasmic granules** and lie in close proximity to free nerve endings. They function as **mechanoreceptors**.

Describe the acute wound healing process.

1. **Coagulation** (immediate): blood clot formation; provides hemostasis and a matrix for cell migration; platelets are the predominant cells.
2. **Inflammation** (days 1-2): monocytes are replaced by neutrophils and function to clear up debris.
3. **Proliferation** and **Migration** (days 3-5): goal is re-epithelialization; granulation occurs during this phase; fibroblasts (secrete collagen framework), pericytes, endothelial cells (aid in angiogenesis), and keratinocytes (responsible for epithelialization) are the major cell types.
4. **Remodeling** (weeks to months): this phase is highly dependent on matrix metalloproteinases and serine proteases; predominant cell type is fibroblast.

Describe the steps involved in wound healing with a skin graft.

1. **Imbibition Phase**: diffusion of plasma into the graft; results in weight increase in graft; phase ends as venous and lymphatic drainage is reestablished and graft weight decreases.
2. **Inosculation Phase**: anastomoses of graft blood vessels with recipient vessels.
3. **Neovascularization**: ingrowth of new blood vessels.

DERMIS AND HYPODERMIS

What layer lies immediately subjacent to the stratum basalis of the epithelium?

Basal lamina

What structures mediate the interaction between the basal lamina and the stratum basalis?

Hemidesmosomes

Describe the epidermal-dermal junction.

Fingerlike dermal projections (papillae) interdigitate with fingerlike epidermal projections (rete ridges). Each papilla is formed on a lymphofibrovascular core.

The dermis is divided into two layers: papillary and reticular. What cellular and connective tissue elements make up the papillary layer?

Connective tissue **proteins** (oxytalan, elaunin, and collagen) and **cells** (mast cells, fibroblasts, and macrophages)

What is the most prominent cell type in the hypodermis?

Hypodermis is considered separate from dermis and contains mostly **adipocytes**.

HAIR

What skin layers make up the hair complex?

1. **Epidermis:** external root sheath
2. **Basal lamina:** glassy membrane
3. **Papillary dermis:** connective tissue

Describe the four phases of hair growth cycle.

1. **Telogen**: phase of quiescence
2. **Anagen**: phase of rapid hair growth; duration varies by region of body and determines final length of hair
3. **Catagen**: apoptosis-driven follicle regression
4. **Exogen**: hair shedding

Unlike the epidermis, cellular differentiation in the hair follicle is neither uniform nor unidirectional. What is the only recognizable epidermal layer in the hair bulb?

Stratum basalis

Blood supply to and drainage from the base of the hair bulb is facilitated by what structures?

Dermal papillae

Hair color is determined by what type of cell?

Melanocyte

What structures, continuous with the external root sheath, can be found in hair follicles?

Sebaceous glands

The development of goose bumps in cold weather is directly controlled by what histologic structure?

Arrector pili muscles are smooth muscle bundles affixed to dermal connective tissue sheaths that contract to produce goose bumps.

How do the secretions of sebaceous glands differ from those of serous glands?

Holocrine secretions (sebaceous): waxy and contain cytoplasmic vesicle contents and cellular debris

Apocrine and merocrine secretions (serous): thin proteinaceous fluids containing only the contents of cytoplasmic vesicles

What are the principal functions of apocrine sweat glands?

Under the control of androgens and estrogens, apocrine glands play a role in the **body scent** of pubertal teens. Under adrenergic stimulation, these glands also produce **pheromones**.

Located in the dermis, sebaceous glands are compound acinar glands with rounded apical cells containing cytoplasmic lipid droplets. What is the function of these glands?

Sebaceous glands are activated by androgens and inhibited by estrogens. During puberty, these glands are active and thought to function in acne development.

Found in the dermis, eccrine (sweat) glands are coiled tubular glands with a myoepithelial capsule, containing clear basal and dark luminal cells with apical secretory granules. How do these glands function? Under cholinergic control, these glands produce watery, merocrine secretions to regulate body temperature, and under adrenergic control, they facilitate emotional sweating.

CLINICAL CORRELATES AND VIGNETTES

A 28 yo M reports progressive skin depigmentation all over his body but particularly over sites sensitive to pressure and friction, where he wears his belt and watch. His dermatologist clinically diagnoses him with segmental vitiligo. What is the pathologic hallmark of vitiligo?

A loss of epidermal melanocytes

A 26 yo blonde construction worker notices a round ulcerating lesion on his nose. The dermatologist describes the lesion as a pearly papule with overlying telangiectases, rolled borders, and central ulceration (see Figure 9.2). What are you most concerned about?

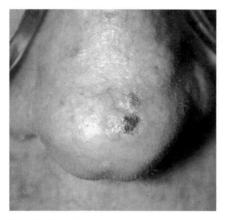

Figure 9.2   Nodular basal cell carcinoma. (*Reproduced, with permission, from Wolff K, Goldsmith LA, Katz SI, et al.* Fitzpatrick's Dermatology in General Medicine. *7th ed. New York,NY: McGraw-Hill; 2007.*)

Nodular basal cell carcinoma. This is the most classic form. Risk factors for basal cell carcinoma include being blonde or red haired, having fair skin, or blue or green eyes; exposures to arsenic, ionizing radiation, smoking, or UV light.

Other types of basal cell carcinoma include

1. Superficial basal cell carcinoma—appears as scaly, erythematous patches or plaques
2. Morpheaform basal cell carcinoma—appears as an indurated, whitish, scar-like plaque.

A 31 yo F reports a h/o chronic, relapsing pruritus that started during childhood. The lesions involve flexures, the nape of the neck, and dorsal aspects of the limbs. She reports during her 20s, the lesions became lichenified plaques. Her PMHx includes asthma. She is diagnosed with atopic dermatitis. What will histology show?

Atopic dermatitis is also known as eczema or "the itch that rashes." It results from a disturbance of the epidermal-barrier function leading to an IgE-mediated sensitization to food or environmental allergens. The histologic features of the plaques are epidermal intercellular edema (spongiosis) and prominent perivascular dermal infiltrates of lymphocytes, monocytes, dendritic cells, and eosinophils.

CHAPTER 10

Digestive System

GENERAL ORGANIZATION

What are the four principal layers of the digestive system from outermost to most luminal?

1. Serosa
2. Muscularis propria
3. Submucosa
4. Mucosa

What three layers make up the mucosa?

1. Epithelium
2. Lamina propria
3. Muscularis mucosa

In a tissue section, how is the lamina propria identified from the other layers and sublayers?

It interdigitates with the luminal epithelium, which in the esophagus and anus forms papillae. It rests on a thin smooth muscle band.

How are the myenteric (Auerbach) and submucosal (Meissner) plexuses different from the autonomic innervation of the gut?

Auerbach and Meissner plexuses constitute the **enteric nervous system**; these ganglia reside inside the gut wall and **function with or without CNS influence**. By contrast autonomic (para- and sympathetic) fibers are extrinsic to the gut and function in a CNS-dependent manner.

What does the submucosal plexus innervate?

Controlling GI secretions, the submucosal plexus innervates intestinal endocrine cells, glands, submucosal blood vessels, and the muscularis mucosa.

What type of innervation does the myenteric plexus supply?

Motor innervation to the muscularis propria and interneuronal communication

Luminal constriction and propulsion are functions of what structures found in the muscularis propria?

Circularly and longitudinally disposed muscles

Secretory IgA is one of the products from what immune system outposts scattered throughout the mucosa and submucosa?

Lymphoid nodules—in the alimentary system, primary lymphocyte aggregates and secondary lymphoid nodules with germinal centers secrete **IgM, IgG**, and primarily **IgA**. In the **oropharynx**, these structures are called **tonsils**, whereas in the **intestine** they are called **Peyer's patches**.

The interstitial cells of Cajal are stellate cells with smooth muscle-like features that reside near the myenteric plexus and interface with the layer of circular muscle. What is the function of those cells?

Those cells function as the **intrinsic pacemaker cells** of the GI tract. They initiate a basic electrical rhythm of spontaneous fluctuations in membrane potential among the smooth muscle cells. When coupled with spike potentials exceeding a depolarization threshold, **smooth muscle contractions, peristalsis**, and **migrating motor complexes** occur.

MOUTH AND PHARYNX

What constitutes the dominant epithelial type in the oropharyngeal portion of the digestive system?

Nonkeratinized, stratified squamous epithelium

What structures, found within the oral mucosa, function to maintain a wet epithelium?

Salivary glands

What is the functional difference between the major and minor salivary glands?

The major salivary glands (parotid, submandibular, and sublingual) are **regulated by the autonomic nervous system in response to environmental cues (secretagogues),** while the minor salivary glands secrete continuously.

How does the parotid gland differ from the submandibular and sublingual glands?

Parotid gland is a **serous** (branched acinar) gland that produces watery secretions.

Submandibular and **sublingual glands** are **mucous** and **serous** (branched tubuloacinar) glands that produce viscous secretions.

Describe the pharyngeal epithelium.

Respiratory epithelium, which is **pseudostratified ciliated columnar epithelium** with **goblet cells**, lines the respiratory portions of the pharynx.

TONGUE

What are the gross structural differences between the anterior two-thirds and posterior one-third of the tongue?

The tongue is composed predominantly of skeletal muscle separated by connective tissue planes. The anterior surface of the tongue has a papillary architecture. The posterior surface of the tongue has a lymphoid architecture.

What are papillae?

Mucosal elevations that function in taste reception and digestion. The four types of papillae are **circumvallate, foliate, fungiform**, and **filiform**.

How is the anterior portion of the tongue divided from the posterior portion?

By a border of circumvallate papillae adopting a V-shape.

What are the nerves of taste, sensation, and motor function of the tongue?

See Table 10.1
See Figure 10.1

Table 10.1 Tongue Innervation

Location on Tongue	Innervation		
	Taste	Sensation	Motor
Anterior two-thirds	CN VII (facial nerve)	Lingual nerve (V3 branch of CN V, trigeminal nerve)	CN XII (hypoglossal nerve)
Posterior one-third	CN IX (glossopharyngeal nerve)	CN IX (glossopharyngeal nerve)	CN XII (hypoglossal nerve)

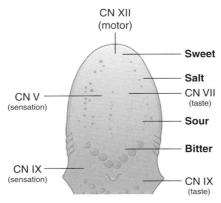

Figure 10.1 Tongue innervation. (*Adapted, with permission, from Waxman SG.* Clinical Neuroanatomy. *26th ed. New York, NY: McGraw-Hill; 2009.*)

ESOPHAGUS AND STOMACH

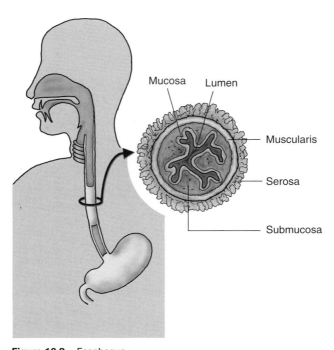

Figure 10.2 Esophagus.

Contrast the upper with lower esophageal sphincter?

Upper esophageal sphincter: formed from horizontal skeletal muscle fibers (cricopharyngeal and inferior pharyngeal constrictor muscles)

Lower esophageal sphincter: composed of both esophageal smooth muscle and skeletal muscle from the crural part of the diaphragm

The muscle forming the upper esophageal sphincter incompletely covers the posterior aspect of the esophagus, leaving the underlying thin, circular layer exposed. What pathologic process can occur in this area?

Absence of the longitudinal muscle layer at this location weakens the esophageal wall, enabling the formation of a sac or outpouching of the esophagus in susceptible individuals. This saccular protrusion of the upper esophagus is called **Zenker's diverticulum**.

What is unique about the muscle histology of the esophagus?

Consists of both **skeletal** and **smooth muscle**

What are the four interconnected layers of veins found in the lower esophageal mucosal folds?

The four venous layers are:
1. **Radially arranged epithelial channels**
2. **Superficial submucosal venous plexuses**
3. **Deep submucosal venous trunks**
4. **Adventitial veins**

In portal hypertension, these veins provide a major shunt for blood returning from the abdomen and lower body. Dilation of this venous system causes esophageal varices and a subsequent rupture can lead to death.

What epithelial transition occurs at the mucosal gastroesophageal junction?

In the lower esophagus, there is a transition from **nonkeratinizing, stratified squamous epithelium to simple columnar epithelium with gastric glands**.

What is Barrett's esophagus?

Metaplastic changes of the lower esophageal epithelium, resulting in a change to intestinal or gastric type adenomatous epithelium. It is secondary to repeat acid exposure, as seen in gastroesophageal reflux disease (GERD). Barrett's esophagus is a strong risk factor for esophageal adenocarcinoma.

How does the muscularis propria of the stomach differ from that of the esophagus and intestine?

Stomach: the muscularis propria consists of **three smooth muscle layers** (inner oblique, middle circular, and outer longitudinal).

Intestine and esophagus: two layers of smooth muscle are present (inner circular and outer longitudinal). Additionally, the esophagus contains striated skeletal muscle.

What are the three histologic and four anatomic regions of the stomach?

Histologic
1. Cardia
2. Fundus
3. Pylorus

Anatomic
1. Cardia
2. Fundus
3. Body
4. Pylorus

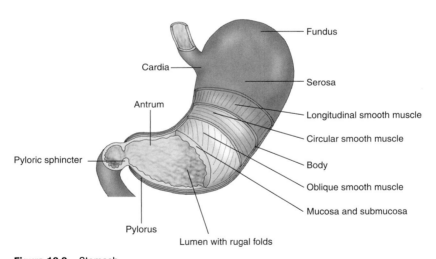

Figure 10.3   Stomach.

How do gastric gland secretions differ among the various histologic regions of the stomach?

Cardiac and pyloric glands: secrete mucus, pepsin, lipase, amylase, and gastrin

Fundic glands: secrete mucus, acid, pepsinogen, and intrinsic factor

Describe how the gastric mucosa can be divided into endocrine and exocrine regions.

See Table 10.2

Table 10.2 Endocrine and Exocrine Regions of the Stomach

Antrum—Endocrine		Fundus—Exocrine	
Hormones secreted into capillaries in the lamina propria		Hormones secreted into gastric ducts and lumen	
Cell Type	Hormone	Cell Type	Hormone
G cells	Gastrin	Chief cells	Pepsinogen
Enterochromaffin cells	Serotonin	Parietal cells	Intrinsic factor
D cells	Somatostatin		

What three mucosal cell types are critical to the normal function of parietal cells and the pathogenesis of gastric ulcers?

1. **Mast cells**
2. **Enterochromaffin-like (ECL) cells**
3. **Parietal cells**

Parietal cells secrete acid into the stomach lumen when stimulated by acetylcholine (vagus nerve), gastrin (G cells), or histamine (mast and ECL cells). In addition to stimulating acid secretion, histamine potentiates the effects of gastrin and acetylcholine on parietal cells. Cimetidine, a histamine H_2 receptor antagonist, and omeprazole, an H^+/K^+-ATPase antagonist, work by blocking parietal cell stimulation and acid secretion, respectively.

Ultrastructurally, in the resting state parietal cells have abundant mitochondria and prominent tubulovesicles, which upon stimulation, transform into an extensive system of tiny canals (canaliculi). What is the function of this ultrastructural transformation?

Acid secretion—when parietal cells are stimulated, vesicles containing membrane-bound H^+/K^+-ATPases (proton pumps) are exocytosed, which traffics the pumps to the cells' luminal surface. Once there, ATP from the abundant mitochondria causes those pumps to acidify the lumen of the stomach. Endocytosis of proton pump–rich regions of the luminal membrane effectively deactivates the pumps.

How do the lymphoid follicles of the stomach differ from those of the rest of the GI system?

Unlike the remainder of the GI tract, the stomach does not usually contain lymphoid follicles. The **presence of lymphoid follicles in the stomach often signifies gastritis** secondary to *Helicobacter pylori* infection.

Contrast chief cells with parietal cells.

Chief cells: granular, basophilic, and located in the base of the gastric glands

Parietal cells: nongranular, acidophilic, and located in the neck and deeper parts of the glands

The pyloric sphincter is formed from a thickening of what muscle layer?

Middle or **circular layer** of the muscularis externa (propria)

SMALL INTESTINE

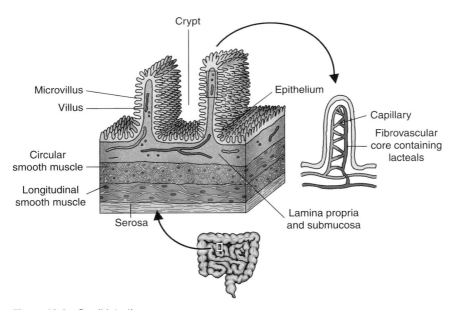

Figure 10.4   Small intestine.

What mucosal structures contribute to the absorption function of the small intestine?

1. Permanent **plicae circulares** increase surface area and slow movement of luminal contents increasing contact time and absorption.
2. **Villi** increase the absorptive surface area.
3. **Microvilli** increase the absorptive surface area, degrade polymers, and take up nutrients.
4. **Lacteals**, or blind ending lymphatic channels, take up fats (**chylomicrons**), cholesterol, and fat-soluble vitamins.
5. **Capillaries** in the lamina propria provide a conduit for absorbed nutrients and minerals.

Functionally, the small intestinal epithelium can be divided into two components. What are those components and their corresponding functions?

1. **Crypt epithelium**—epithelial renewal
2. **Villous epithelium**—absorption

Segments of the small intestine can be differentiated on gross observation by what feature?

Density of the plicae circulares (or Kerckring valves); their prominence is greatest in the jejunum and least in the flanking duodenum and ileum.

What are the cellular components and their respective functions in the small intestinal epithelium?

1. **Enterocytes**—absorption
2. **Goblet cells**—mucus production
3. **M cells**—luminal protein antigen transport to lymphocytes (found only in Peyer's patches in the ileum)
4. **Stem cells**—epithelial renewal
5. **Paneth cells**—defense against microbes (lysozyme and α-defensins)
6. **Enteroendocrine cells**—hormones regulating GI function

How do I, S, K, and Mo cells function in the upper portion of the small intestine?   See Table 10.3

Table 10.3 Functions of Enteroendocrine Cell Types

Enteroendocrine cell type	I cells	S cells	K cells	Mo cells
Hormone secretion	Cholecystokinin (CCK)	Secretin	Gastrin inhibitory peptide (GIP)	Motilin
Function of hormone or protein	Stimulates pancreatic and biliary secretions and works with secretin to stimulate pancreatic bicarbonate secretion	Stimulates bicarbonate release to buffer gastric acid in the duodenum	Stimulates insulin release from pancreatic β cells and inhibits gastrin secretion	Stimulates smooth muscle contraction during fasting creating migratory motor complexes

What are the three main histologic features of absorptive cells?

1. Tall columnar absorptive cells
2. Basal nuclei
3. Microvilli with brush border digestive enzymes

Protein allergies can involve malabsorption and diarrhea, skin eruptions, and shock in severe cases. What gut epithelial cells are associated with protein allergy development?

Because of their ability to transport protein antigens, **microfold** or **M cells** help sensitize intestinal lymphocytes to luminal antigens, which can lead to an allergic response upon reexposure to that protein antigen. **M cells** overlie Peyer's patches and pass luminal antigens to resident lymphocytes only in the ileum.

LARGE INTESTINE

How does the intestinal epithelium change when moving from the small to large intestine?

Epithelium changes from a predominantly nutrient absorbing epithelium with transporters for many types of biomolecules to:

1. a desiccating epithelium that absorbs Na^+ actively and water passively
2. an epithelium that actively secretes K^+ and HCO^{3-}

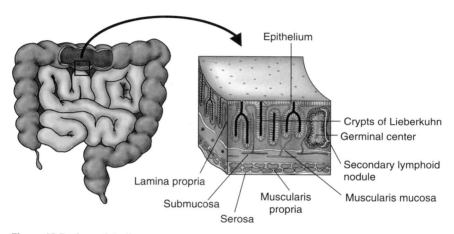

Epithelium

Crypts of Lieberkuhn

Germinal center

Secondary lymphoid nodule

Muscularis mucosa

Muscularis propria

Serosa

Submucosa

Lamina propria

Figure 10.5   Large intestine.

How do large intestinal glands differ from those of the small intestine?

Loss of lysozyme-producing Paneth cells

What three epithelial changes occur in the rectum as the anus emerges?

1. Mucosa assumes **folded appearance** (rectal columns of Morgagni).
2. Simple columnar epithelium becomes **stratified squamous epithelium**.
3. **Large venous plexuses** appear in the rectal mucosa.

VERMIFORM APPENDIX

Appendicitis is an acute inflammatory process of the appendix that can lead to appendiceal rupture. What prominent, normal, histologic trait of the appendix contributes to the development of appendicitis?

Abundant, circumferential lymphoid tissue in the lamina propria contributes to the genesis of appendicitis by causing significant luminal narrowing and mucosal distortion. Fecal material, lymphocyte proliferation, and leukocyte infiltration can easily block this narrow lumen, and failure to clear the blockage can lead to appendiceal inflammation.

Considering the abundant lymphoid tissue present there, what is a potential function of the appendix?

The appendix is a space where fecal material can be sampled and B- and T- lymphocytes can be developed against luminal antigens. These lymphocytes subsequently migrate to other parts of the GI system to enhance **mucosal immune surveillance**.

Carcinoids are neuroendocrine tumors that occur in the GI tract and lungs. What normal feature in appendiceal histology predisposes the appendix to carcinoid tumors?

Appendiceal lamina propria has a well-developed **nervous plexus** containing **abundant endocrine (neurosecretory) cells.** Part of the intrinsic nervous system, these serotonin-producing cells affect communication between Meissner and Auerbach plexuses and the epithelium. Appendiceal carcinoids appear to arise from these cells.

CLINICAL CORRELATES AND VIGNETTES

A 52 yo obese M with a 20-yr history of untreated GERD visits his physician with complaints of black stools, worsening abdominal pain, and cough. Upon endoscopic exam, his lower esophagus looks like gastric epithelium, with multiple friable masses. On biopsy, the tissue appears disorganized, with numerous goblet-like cells and almost no ordered superstructure. What is the most likely diagnosis, and what caused it?

Friable adenomatous tissue in the lower esophagus suggests **esophageal adenocarcinoma**. Given the history, it is likely that this patient had **Barrett's esophagus** secondary to unmanaged GERD. GERD causes Barrett's by reactive metaplasia of the lower esophageal epithelium in response to the presence of gastric acid. Controlling acid secretion with PPI or H_2 receptor blockers prevents the development of Barrett's. The only management for esophageal adenocarcinoma is resection.

A 15 yo Jewish M c/o malodorous, fatty stools and intense abdominal pain. He also c/o recent onset of incontinence. On exam, his rectal tone is normal, but there is a fistulous tract draining from his large intestine to his perineum. Colonoscopy reveals discontinuous ulcerated regions in his transverse colon. What is the diagnosis, and what cytokine is responsible for his pathology?

Discontinuous ulcerated lesions suggest **Crohn's disease**. Fistulous tracts can occur during inflammatory bowel diseases. Fistulae that occur with Crohn's are often reversible with anti-TNFα therapy (such as infliximab or adalimumab), the cytokine thought to be integral to Crohn's.

A 74 yo uninsured F c/o weight loss despite increased oral intake, abdominal pain, intermittent constipation, and bright red blood per rectum. Because of affordability of care issues, she has never had a colonoscopy. On abdominal exam, there is a palpable LLQ mass. What diagnosis should you be concerned about? If she develops gram-positive bacteremia, what is the likely species?

The case is concerning for **colorectal cancer.** Approximately 15% of people with colorectal cancer will go on to develop *Streptococcus bovis* bacteremia.

CHAPTER 11

Hepatobiliary System

PANCREAS

What is the general organization of the pancreas?

Contains both exocrine and endocrine tissue. Islands of endocrine cell cords abutting fenestrated capillaries are scattered throughout a sea of acinar exocrine glands containing pyramidal cells with prominent zymogen granules.

When acidic chyme is released into the small intestine, on what pancreatic tissue does secretin and cholecystokinin work to help neutralize the chyme and degrade the biopolymers therein?

Secretin stimulates **ductal cells** to secrete bicarbonate-rich fluid to neutralize the chyme. **Cholecystokinin** stimulates **acinar cell degranulation**. Those granules contain digestive proenzymes (zymogens) activated in the small intestinal lumen.

LIVER

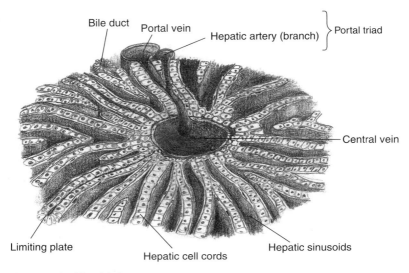

Figure 11.1   Liver lobules.

What are the six major cell types found in the liver and their functions?

1. **Hepatocytes**—substrate synthesis, processing, secretion, degradation, and oxidation
2. **Kupffer cells**—phagocytosis and acute inflammation; line the sinusoids
3. **Endothelial cells**—regulate filtration of the portal venous circulation, and inflammation; line the sinusoids
4. **Ductal epithelial cells**—bile conduction
5. **Hepatic stellate (Ito) cells**—fat and vitamin A storage; extracellular matrix production and degradation; causes fibrosis in cirrhosis
6. **Pit cells**—lymphocytes with natural killer cell activity; viral and malignancy surveillance; line the sinusoids

Three models are used to describe liver organization: the classic lobule, the portal lobule, and liver acinus models. Describe those models and give their functional significance:

1. **Classic lobule model:** This model emphasizes the endocrine function. It is based on thearrangement of the branches of the portal vein and hepatic artery (thepath of blood flow as it perfuses the hepatocytes). The boundaries of the classic lobules are defined by connective tissue septa from the capsule.
2. **Portal lobule model:** The portal lobule model emphasizes the exocrine function of the liver, namely bile secretion. The portal bile duct is at the center. Its outer margins are imaginary lines drawn between three central veins that are closest to that portal triad.
3. **Liver acinus model:** This model has at its center the blood supply (portal and arterial) to the liver parenchyma, rather than its venous drainage; emphasizes oxygen and nutrient gradient. This model describes the smallest functional unit in the liver parenchyma.

Give the functional significance of zone 1 cells in the acinar model:

The ovoid hepatic acinus model centers on the portal triad (trunk) and projects acinar sinusoids (branches) to terminal hepatic veins. Cells in the liver acinus are arranged into three concentric, elliptical zones.

Zone 1 cells: closest to distributing arteries and veins

They are the first to:
1. be affected by or to alter the incoming blood
2. receive both nutrients and toxins
3. take up glucose to store as glycogen after a meal
4. break down glycogen in response to fasting
5. show morphological changes following bile duct occlusion

If circulation is impaired, they are the last to die and the first to regenerate.

Give the functional significance of zone 3 cells in the acinar model:

Zone 3 cells: farthest from the distributing vessels and closest to the central vein

1. They are the first to show ischemic necrosis and fat accumulation
2. They are the last to respond to toxic substances and bile stasis.

Describe the sinusoid and its supporting "basement membrane." How does this histologic organization affect filtration into the liver parenchyma?

Portal sinusoids consist of a layer of endothelial and Kupffer cells supported by a thin reticular (collagen III) fiber network. There is no basement membrane to filter any material flowing out of the sinusoids. Rather, the sinusoids are lined by a fenestrated epithelium high in endocytic capacity, which filters the material as it passes through them.

What is the space of Disse, and how does it function?

It is the interstitial space between the portal sinusoids and the cords of hepatocytes. Materials are exchanged here between neighboring hepatocytes and the blood, and fluid is filtered from the space of Disse to the lymphatic channels.

What are the four components of the "triad"?

1. Bile duct
2. Hepatic artery
3. Portal vein (classic triad)
4. Lymphatic channels

What is the Glisson capsule?

Layer of connective tissue surrounding the liver and the portal triad as it branches within the liver.

What is the clinical significance of the Glisson capsule?

In disease, blood and tumors (eg, adenocarcinoma) amass right underneath the intact capsule and do not spill into the peritoneal cavity.

What is the limiting plate?

A distinct border formed by a row of conjoined hepatocytes surrounding the portal tracts. Inflammatory cell infiltration and destruction of this structure in chronic hepatitis leads to **piecemeal necrosis**.

What are the apical, basal, and lateral surfaces of the polyhedral hepatocyte?

Apical: bile canaliculus

Basal: sinusoids

Lateral: junctional complexes

Hepatocytes produce many blood proteins; yet, unlike other protein exporting cells, they have no cytoplasmic secretory granules. Why not?

Hepatocytes continually release proteins into the blood; therefore, secretory granules never build up in the cytoplasm.

GALLBLADDER

Deep infections and inflammation of the gallbladder wall are facilitated by what normal structures?

Rokitansky-Aschoff sinuses. These structures are epithelial herniations into the lamina propria, submucosal smooth muscle, and subserosal perimuscular connective tissue. In susceptible individuals, infectious microorganisms may use these sinuses to access deep layers of the gallbladder wall.

Cholesterol stones are fairly common among obese women older than 40 years who use oral contraceptives in the United States. What component of the gallbladder epithelium contributes strongly to gallstone development?

Na^+ pumps in the microvilli of the simple columnar epithelium stimulate passive intercellular water absorption. Of the three factors involved in cholesterol stone formation (bile stasis, bile supersaturation with cholesterol, and nucleation factors), these epithelial pumps contribute to this process by desiccating stored bile and disturbing the balance between the relative concentrations of cholesterol and bile salts.

What hormone interacts with submucosal smooth muscle to facilitate gallbladder contraction?

Cholecystokinin

What structures prevent gallstones from damaging the gallbladder epithelium but also assist in gallstone formation?

Tubuloacinar glands found in the lamina propria secrete mucus, which protects the gallbladder epithelium from potential damaging effects of gallstones. This mucus also provides the environment for cholesterol crystals to grow into gallstones.

CLINICAL CORRELATES AND VIGNETTES

A 24 yo M develops jaundice 2 weeks after returning from a hiking trip in the rain forests of Brazil. He reports that he often wandered in open shoes, occasionally wading through shallow streams. He recalls one episode of having "itchy ankles" and noticing "red dots" that resolved over a few weeks. Labs reveal a marked eosinophilia and normal ESR and CRP. What is the likely diagnosis? Why is he jaundiced?

Eosinophilia in a young otherwise healthy person in the context of foreign travel should raise concerns for parasitic infection. *Schistosoma mansoni* or "liver flukes" are transmitted through the skin in shallow waters. Males and females of the species anchor themselves in the mesenteric portal circulation, and their eggs saturate and obstruct clearance of the liver, leading to hepatic necrosis.

A 44 yo obese F with 4 children complains of intermittent pain underneath her right scapula that is exacerbated after eating fatty foods. She has a h/o gallstones but has not had a cholecystectomy. What is the likely diagnosis?

In this vignette, the patient follows the "four F" rule—female, fertile, fat, over forty—characteristics known to elevate the risk of gallstones. The location of the pain and precipitation with fatty meals suggests **biliary colic,** a process in which gallstones obstruct the biliary tree at the gallbladder neck. This increases the back pressure in the gallbladder and leads to pain that resolves once the stones shift and the biliary tree is once again clear. Because the pain is intermittent, no gallstones are lodged within the biliary tree, as this would produce a constant pain.

A 32 yo M p/w abdominal pain, weight loss, and painless jaundice, and reports greasy stools and dark urine. On exam, a palpable gallbladder is felt at the right costal margin. On CT scan, there is a pancreatic mass, dilatation of the biliary system, and pancreatic duct. You order an ERCP to obtain brushings for cytology. What type of cells do you expect to see?

The majority of pancreatic cancers are adenocarcinomas arising from the ductal epithelium. On cytology, malignant ductal cells will most likely be seen. The palpable gallbladder exam finding is c/w **Courvoisier sign**, strongly indicative of pancreatic cancer.

CHAPTER 12

Urinary System

KIDNEY ORGANIZATION

What organizing structures of the kidneys are present when viewed in gross section?

The two main components of the kidneys include the **outer cortex** and **inner medulla**, which contains the **medullary pyramids** and **rays**. Other grossly visible structures include the major and minor **calyces** and **renal pelvis**.

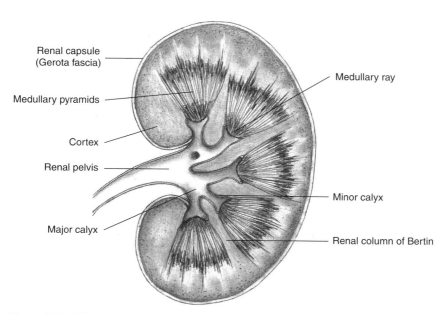

Renal capsule (Gerota fascia)

Medullary pyramids

Cortex

Renal pelvis

Major calyx

Medullary ray

Minor calyx

Renal column of Bertin

Figure 12.1   Kidney.

The nephron is the basic functional unit of the kidneys. What are the constituent parts of the nephron?

Renal corpuscle and **renal tubules** (proximal tubule, loop of Henle, and distal tubule)

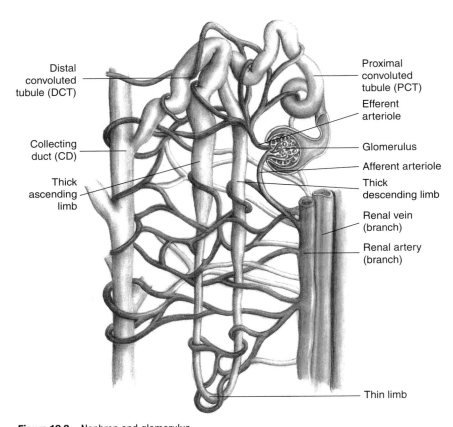

Distal convoluted tubule (DCT)

Collecting duct (CD)

Thick ascending limb

Proximal convoluted tubule (PCT)

Efferent arteriole

Glomerulus

Afferent arteriole

Thick descending limb

Renal vein (branch)

Renal artery (branch)

Thin limb

Figure 12.2   Nephron and glomerulus.

What parts of the nephron and collecting duct (CD) system are located in the renal cortex, medulla, and medullary rays?

Cortex—renal corpuscles, proximal, and distal convoluted tubules (DCTs)

Medulla—loop of Henle (thick and thin descending, thick ascending)

Medullary rays—collecting ducts

RENAL CORPUSCLE

The renal corpuscle filters the blood and collects the filtrate in the urinary space. Which two components of the renal corpuscle are responsible for this function?

1. The **filtering unit** or **glomerulus** is composed of a capillary tuft, its subjacent basement membrane, and filtration slits formed by interdigitating podocyte foot processes (visceral Bowman's capsule).
2. The **collecting unit** or **parietal Bowman's capsule** is composed of a simple squamous epithelium, its subjacent basal lamina, and reticular fibers.

Filtration at the glomerulus selects molecules based on ionic charges and sizes less than 8 nm in diameter. Among similarly sized molecules, those with a net positive charge are filtered more readily than those with a net neutral or negative charge. How do the three components of the glomerulus contribute to this selective permeability?

1. The **capillary endothelium** contains membrane pores (fenestrations) and negatively charged sialoproteins, which contribute the first level of size and charge selectivity.
2. The **glomerular basement membrane** contains collagen IV and negatively charged heparan sulfate, which adds a second level of charge selectivity.
3. The **filtration slits** are covered by a thin membrane, which adds another layer of size selectivity.

What is a podocyte?

A round cell projecting primary processes to nearby blood vessels from which secondary (or foot) processes extend. These lateral secondary processes, also called pedicels, oppose the glomerular basement membrane and interdigitate to form filtration slits.

How are podocytes affected in minimal change disease?

Large amounts of protein are lost in the urine (**proteinuria**) because the **foot processes are damaged** and are not replaced. It is one of the most common causes of the nephrotic syndrome.

What are mesangial cells, and how do they affect filtration at the glomerulus?

They are stellate, contractile smooth muscle-like cells that adhere to glomerular capillary walls and secrete the connective tissue (mesangium), which holds the glomerulus together. Mesangial cells have receptors for angiotensin II (vasoconstrictor) and atrial natriuretic factor (vasodilator). These cells can reduce or increase glomerular filtration by controlling the effective capillary surface area available for filtration.

How are mesangial cells affected in IgA nephropathy?

IgA is deposited in the mesangium resulting in hematuria.

Inulin is used to determine the glomerular filtration rate because it is filtered at the glomerulus, but not reabsorbed or secreted in the tubules. A molecule of inulin filtered through the glomerulus lies in what area?

Urinary space of Disse

PROXIMAL CONVOLUTED TUBULE (PCT)

The PCT resorbs all glucose and amino acids as well as 85% of the NaCl and water filtered at the glomerulus. What features of proximal tubular cells facilitate its extensive reabsorptive capacity?

The proximal tubule contains simple columnar cells with abundant microvilli **(brush border)** and **lateral intercellular spaces**. The brush border contains numerous transmembrane proteins that enable sodium-coupled, secondary active nutrient reabsorption, passive water reabsorption along the osmotic gradient, receptor-mediated endocytosis of filtered proteins, and active solute reabsorption. The **lateral interstitial spaces** provide "reservoirs" for a sodium-rich fluid that will either be reabsorbed by peritubular capillaries or leak into the tubular lumen.

Glomerulotubular balance is a process by which changes in glomerular filtration elicit an immediate compensatory response in proximal tubular reabsorption. For example, an increase in glomerular filtration causes a concomitant increase in solute reabsorption at the proximal tubule. What structures facilitate this process?

Peritubular capillaries enable glomerulotubular balance. As glomerular filtration increases, it generates a high intravascular plasma oncotic pressure, which drives increased nutrient reabsorption in the peritubular capillaries.

What other proximal tubular function is facilitated by the presence of leaky peritubular capillaries?

Proximal tubules actively secrete substances received from peritubular capillaries into the lumen for urinary excretion.

LOOP OF HENLE

In the U-shaped loop of Henle, thick and thin refers to what histologic phenomenon?

Epithelium types—thick refers to a simple cuboidal epithelium, whereas thin refers to a simple squamous epithelium

What structural feature of the loop facilitates the concentration of urine?

Length—the loop of Henle establishes a solute gradient that increases deep within the medullary pyramids. Since this solute gradient facilitates the concentration of urine, the longer the loop, the better the ability of the nephron to concentrate urine.

Countercurrent multiplication establishes the osmolality gradient along the medullary pyramids, and thereby concentrates the urine. What property of the loop of Henle enables countercurrent multiplication and the formation of concentrated urine?

Differing permeabilities along each limb enable countercurrent multiplication.

1. The descending thin limb is freely permeable to water and impermeable to solutes creating a hypertonic filtrate.
2. The entire ascending limb is impermeable to water, yet permeable to sodium, chloride, and potassium (in the thick segment) creating a hypotonic filtrate.

This sequence concentrates, then dilutes tubular fluid, and increases the osmolality (solute) gradient in the medullary interstitium.

While countercurrent multiplication is necessary to establish the solute gradient, a countercurrent exchange mechanism is needed to maintain this gradient. What structures are involved in maintaining the solute gradient?

Vasa rectae are large capillary networks that envelop the loop of Henle and maintain the solute gradient by the countercurrent exchange mechanism. NaCl and urea diffuse from the ascending to the descending limb of this network while water diffuses in the opposite direction. Consequently, water bypasses deeper hyperosmolar segments of the medullary pyramids, whereas solutes cycle within the pyramids and maintain the solute gradient.

In addition to cell size, what fundamental functional difference exists between the thick and thin ascending limbs of the Henle loop?

NaCl transport out of the thin ascending limb occurs passively along the concentration gradients and is facilitated by transmembrane channels. NaCl and KCl transport out of the thick ascending limb is an active process requiring transmembrane pumps.

DISTAL CONVOLUTED TUBULE (DCT)

The DCT contacts the vascular pole of the renal corpuscle. At this contact point, both the DCT and the afferent arteriole are modified to form the juxtaglomerular apparatus. What is this apparatus, and what is its function?

It is a cell complex formed by renin-producing juxtaglomerular (JG) cells, mesangial cells, and the macula densa. Mesangial cells and the macula densa function in the tubuloglomerular feedback mechanism. JG cells release renin, a protein hormone that activates the angiotensin-aldosterone system by cleaving angiotensinogen to angiotensin I, when stimulated by sympathetic neurons or local baroreceptors. It functions in blood pressure maintenance and total body Na+ and K+ balance.

COLLECTING DUCT

The collecting duct can generally be divided into three functional regions—the cortical, outer medullary, and inner medullary collecting ducts. What functions are associated with these regions?

Cortical collecting duct — K^+, HCO_3^- secretion and Na^+, HCO_3^- reabsorption

Outer medullary collecting duct — urine acidification (H^+ secretion) and K^+ reabsorption

Inner medullary collecting duct — urine concentration via water and urea reabsorption

What are principal cells?

Hormone-sensitive cuboidal cells that reabsorb sodium and water through independent processes

What are intercalated cells?

Cuboidal cells with abundant apical microplicae (luminal folds) and microvilli. These cells function in urine acidification, bicarbonate secretion and reabsorption, and K^+ reabsorption.

How does removing urea from luminal fluid in the inner medullary collecting duct aid in concentrating the urine?

Urea, reabsorbed through urea transporters in the terminal collecting ducts, is ultimately transported into the medullary pyramids where it contributes to the maintenance of the inner medullary osmolality gradient. This gradient enables the loop of Henle to concentrate urine.

What glycoprotein hormone is released from interstitial cells in the peritubular capillary beds in response to hypoxia?

Erythropoietin (EPO) acts on erythroid bone marrow stem cells to promote differentiation into red blood cells (RBCs). Symptomatic anemia is a common complication of chronic renal failure.

URINARY PASSAGE AND BLADDER

What is transitional epithelium, and where is it found?

Stratified sheet of cuboidal cells with scalloped, cerebroside-rich apical membranes. It is found in the calyces, renal pelvis, ureters, and bladder.

What is the general histologic organization of the ureters and bladder?

It is lined by transitional epithelium, with underlying loose and dense connective tissue (lamina propria), and three layers of smooth muscle (spiral, circular, and longitudinal). Activation of smooth muscle stretch receptors stimulates reflexive contraction, peristalsis in the ureters, and contraction of the bladder.

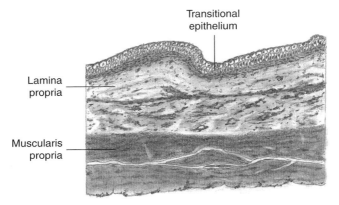

Figure 12.3 Histology of the bladder.

CLINICAL CORRELATES AND VIGNETTES

A 23 yo F with recurrent urinary tract infections p/w 2 days of fever and urinary hesitancy, urgency, and increased frequency. PE reveals right-side flank pain. Her urine analysis reveals white blood cell casts. What would a renal biopsy reveal?

Acute pyelonephritis is histologically characterized by numerous neutrophils filling the renal tubules. Leukocytes in the distal renal tubules and collecting ducts may be flushed out appearing as white cell casts in the urine.

A 27 yo M c/o puffiness around his eyes and ankles. Lab results confirm your suspicions of nephrotic syndrome, showing hypoalbuminemia, hyperlipidemia, and proteinuria. What is the histopathology of this patient's proteinuria and hypoalbuminemia?

Nephrotic syndrome is a nonspecific disorder characterized by edema, hyperlipidemia, hypoalbuminemia, proteinuria, and hypertension. Podocyte effacement in the kidneys allows protein to leak into the urine, causing hypoalbuminemia in the blood. This loss of oncotic pressure causes a fluid shift, resulting in edema. Histologic classifications of nephrotic syndrome include minimal change disease, focal segmental glomerular sclerosis, membranous nephropathy, and membranoproliferative glomerular nephropathy.

An 80 yo M in the ICU has fever, hypotension, and altered mental status, consistent with severe sepsis. The following morning urine output is only 150 cc. What would microscopic examination of the urine show?

This case is consistent with ischemic **acute tubular necrosis (ATN)**, a serious condition in which hypotension leads to tubular cell death and acute renal failure. Muddy brown casts of the necrotic proximal tubules are shed into the urine.

CHAPTER 13

Reproductive Systems

OVARY

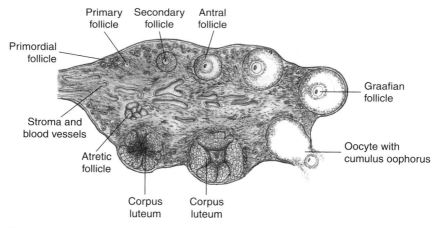

Primary follicle
Secondary follicle
Antral follicle
Primordial follicle
Graafian follicle
Stroma and blood vessels
Oocyte with cumulus oophorus
Atretic follicle
Corpus luteum
Corpus luteum

Figure 13.1 Ovary.

What are the two main functions of the ovary?

1. Production of female gametes (ova) through oogenesis
2. Production of steroid sex hormones

What structures and hormones are involved in the hypothalamic-pituitary-ovarian axis?

Begins in the hypothalamic arcuate nucleus with gonadotropin-releasing hormone (GnRH) release. Pulsatile GnRH stimulates anterior pituitary release of follicle-stimulating hormone (FSH) and luteinizing hormone (LH), which causes the ovaries to release estrogen and progesterone. Negative feedback regulates FSH and LH.

What is the histologic structure of the ovary beginning from outside to inside?

The ovarian surface is a simple cuboidal epithelium, which is continuous with the peritoneal mesothelium. Underneath lies the tunica albuginea (superficial cortex), a thin fibrous connective tissue capsule. The ovary then comprises an outer cortex, containing numerous follicles in various stages of development, and an inner medulla, composed of loose connective tissue, blood and lymphatic vessels, and nerves.

Ovarian follicle generation is a continuous process where follicle maturation begins in the luteal phase, continues into the follicular phase, and ends at ovulation. What are the five ovarian follicle types, in the order of maturity?

1. Primordial
2. Primary
3. Pre-antral
4. Antral
5. Mature (graafian) follicles

Describe the primordial follicle.

Spherical oocyte surrounded by a layer of squamous granulosa cells resting on a thin basement membrane. The oocyte is arrested in the diplotene stage of meiosis I, while the granulosa cells are mitotically inactive.

How do primary and secondary follicles differ from each other?

Primary follicles: granulosa cells have just resumed gonadotropin-independent mitosis and thus form a single layer of cuboidal cells around the oocyte.

Secondary follicles: mitotically active granulosa cells proliferate to form a stratified layer and secrete a glycoprotein-rich capsule (zona pellucida) around the oocyte.

Stimulation by LH causes stromal cells neighboring secondary follicles to differentiate into thecal cells, which subsequently stratify to form the theca interna and externa. How do luteinized thecal cells function in antral follicle development?

According to the two-cell hypothesis, LH-stimulated thecal cells supply androstenedione and testosterone to FSH-stimulated granulosa cells for aromatization to estrone and estradiol, respectively. While both theca and granulosa cells are needed to supply plasma estrogens, granulosa cells concentrate supraphysiologic levels of follicular fluid estrogens for follicle growth and maturation.

Luteinization is a process of steroidogenic vesicle development in ovarian cells. Stimulated by LH, granulosa and thecal cells undergo luteinization and form what ovarian structure?

Corpus luteum

How does the corpus luteum of pregnancy differ from the corpus luteum of menstruation?

Corpus luteum of menstruation: active for the first 10 to 14 days after ovulation. In the absence of fertilization and implantation, it ceases to produce progesterone and estrogen, and degenerates into a white scar, called the corpus albicans.

Corpus luteum of pregnancy: placental human chorionic somatomammotropin (hCG) stimulates and maintains the corpus luteum of pregnancy until the 12th week. After that point, the placenta becomes the primary source of hormones until parturition.

FALLOPIAN TUBES

What are the four regions of the fallopian tube, and what functional significance does each segment possess?

1. **Infundibulum**—the funnel-shaped, lateral end of the tube, with fingerlike projections (fimbriae) sweep over and pick up the ovum immediately after ovulation
2. **Ampulla**—the largest tubular segment (diameter), where fertilization usually occurs
3. **Isthmus**—the narrowest tubular segment, lying lateral to the uterus
4. **Interstitial (intramural)**—penetrates the wall of the uterus and opens into the endometrial cavity

The histologic organization of the fallopian tube is a simple, ciliated columnar epithelium with secretory cells, a subjacent lamina propria, and a muscularis with inner circular and outer longitudinal smooth muscle. Considering this organization, which attribute of fallopian tube histology functions in secondary oocyte transport into the uterine cavity?

Ciliary motion contributes more readily to the movement of the egg to the fertilization site within the ampulla of the fallopian tube.

How does the fallopian tube epithelium change between the follicular and luteal phases of the menstrual cycle?

Follicular phase: circulating estrogens stimulate **ciliogenesis** and increase their growth into the labyrinthine fallopian tube lumen.

Luteal phase: marked by progesterone-induced **regression of epithelial cilia** and an increased number of secretory cells.

UTERUS

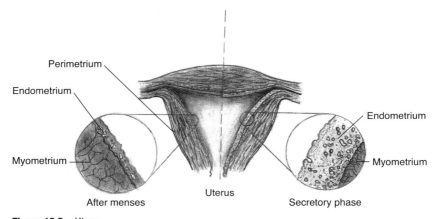

Figure 13.2   Uterus.

The three layers of the uterine body wall are the perimetrium (serosa), myometrium, and endometrium. What is the histologic organization of those three layers?

1. **Perimetrium (serosa)**—the outer uterine layer containing connective tissue and simple squamous mesothelium (parietal peritoneum)
2. **Myometrium**—the middle uterine layer containing two sublayers of longitudinal smooth muscle form a sandwich around a thick, highly vascular layer of circular smooth muscle
3. **Endometrium**—the innermost lining of the uterine cavity is composed of simple columnar epithelium of ciliated and secretory cells, a basal lamina, and a subjacent vascular connective tissue stroma. It is divided into two zones: a superficial, glandular functional epithelium and a deep, regenerative basal stroma.

How do the basal and functional layers of the endometrium differ histologically?

The basal layer proliferates to regenerate the endometrial lining after menses; it contains stem cells, straight arteries, and the basal portions of glands. The functional layer is sloughed off during the menstrual cycle and contains ciliated and secretory epithelial cells, coiled arteries, and tubular glands.

The menstrual cycle consists of three phases based on endometrial appearance—menses, proliferative phase, and secretory phase. A proliferative endometrium contains rapidly dividing, minimally tortuous glands and vessels. A secretory endometrium, however, contains prominent coiled (sawtooth) glands, spiral arteries, maximal stromal edema, and serous glandular secretions. What is the purpose of these changes, and what hormones induce them?

Stimulated solely by estrogens, a proliferative endometrium restores the uterine epithelium shed in the previous menses; a secretory endometrium, stimulated by estrogens and progestins, prepares the uterus for implantation of a fertilized ovum.

How does the endometrium formed during an anovulatory cycle differ from that formed in an ovulatory cycle?

Anovulatory cycles do not generate a corpus luteum, the only progestin source for the uterus. The endometrium continues to proliferate under the effects of unopposed estrogens and never experiences the secretory changes that occur during ovulatory (corpus luteum-generating) cycles. Consequently, the continuously proliferative endometrium becomes too thick, breaks down, and causes irregular menses.

Premenarche is the period before the onset of uterine bleeding during puberty, while postmenopause is the period occurring after the last menstrual period. How is the premenarchal endometrium similar to the postmenopausal endometrium?

In the absence of estrogen stimulation, as in the premenarchal and postmenopausal periods, the endometrium is thin and atrophic with inactive glands and stroma. Menarche and menopause are two periods of irregular uterine bleeding because the endometrium is slowly becoming acclimated to the changing hormonal environment. At menarche, cycles are usually anovulatory.

How does the myometrium of a pregnant (gravid) uterus differ from that of a nonpregnant uterus?

The myometrium of the uterus from a pregnant woman is **thicker** (due to both hypertrophy and hyperplasia) and more **collagenized** compared to the uterus of a woman who is not pregnant.

What are the histologic effects of estrogen and progesterone on the myometrium?

Estrogen stimulates myometrial growth by hyperplasia and hypertrophy and stimulates increased collagen and elastin deposition in the uterus.

Progesterone has no histologic effects; rather, it is believed to inhibit uterine smooth muscle contraction.

CERVIX

Two of the main functions of the cervix are to help maintain pregnancy during the gestational months and facilitate the delivery of the fetus during parturition. How does the structure of the cervix contribute to those functions?

Unlike the uterine body, the cervix contains abundant tough collagenous and elastic fibers but little smooth muscle. The lack of smooth muscle limits cervical expansion and helps maintain pregnancy during the gestational months. In a process called **cervical ripening,** the cervix weakens in response to estrogen-induced collagenases and dilates to facilitate the delivery of the fetus during parturition.

What two epithelial types are found in the cervix?

1. Inner simple columnar epithelium with branched tubular mucous glands and ciliated and cervical mucus-secreting cells
2. Outer stratified squamous epithelium—a transformation zone lies between those two epithelia and marks the transition from one epithelial type to the other. The outer stratified squamous cervical epithelium gives rise to cervical cancer in susceptible individuals.

Unlike the endometrium, the cervical epithelium does not experience cyclical sloughing. However, its mucus-secreting cells are responsive to circulating estrogens and progestins. What effect do cyclical hormonal changes have on mucus production and function?

Cervical mucus blocks microbial entry into the uterus and, depending on the hormonal environment, it either inhibits or enables sperm passage into the uterus and fallopian tubes for fertilization. Estrogen makes cervical mucus thin and alkaline, facilitating sperm maturation and passage into the uterus, while progesterone thickens cervical mucus making it hostile to sperm.

What are Nabothian cysts?

Dilated cysts within the cervix caused by blockage of the openings of the mucosal glands and retention of their mucus secretions. These cysts occur frequently and are benign.

VAGINA

The vaginal mucosa contains a stratified squamous epithelium with an elastic fiber-rich lamina propria that is responsive to ovarian hormonal fluctuation. How does the preovulatory vaginal mucosa differ from the postovulatory mucosa?

Under the influence of estrogen, during the follicular phase, the epithelial cells synthesize and accumulate glycogen as they move toward the surface. With over 45 layers, the epithelium is thickest at this point. In contrast, high postovulatory progestin levels inhibit epithelial proliferation and maturation enabling mucosal thinning.

Vaginal mucosa is usually moist and acidic (pH 4-5). Lactic acid fermentation by resident lactobacilli maintains the acidic pH. What structures provide lubrication for the vaginal surface, and what substrate do lactobacilli use to produce lactic acid?

Lubrication is mainly provided by mucus produced by the cervical glands and the greater and lesser vestibular glands that are located in the wall of the vaginal vestibule. Lactobacilli metabolize glycogen released into the lumen into lactic acid.

The vagina expands during intercourse and constricts after coitus to retain a collection of semen for fertilization. It must also distend grossly to deliver the fetus at parturition. What histologic features of the vaginal wall contribute to its elasticity and strength?

The **muscular layer** is composed of longitudinal and circular smooth muscle that contributes to the constricting properties of the vagina. Surrounding the muscular layer is an adventitial layer that contains a **highly elastic lamina propria**. This component allows the distention needed for vaginal delivery of the fetus.

What vestigial structures found bilaterally in the wall of the vagina can occasionally become filled with fluid leading to cyst formation?

Gartner ducts are remnants of the mesonephric (wolffian) ducts, which degenerate in the female fetus in the absence of testosterone.

Diethylstilbestrol (DES) is a nonsteroidal estrogen that was used in 1938 to prevent miscarriages in high-risk pregnancies. However, in 1971, DES use was discontinued because of its association with the development of what condition in the female offspring of mothers treated with DES during the first trimester?

Clear cell adenocarcinoma of the vagina and cervix

MAMMARY GLANDS

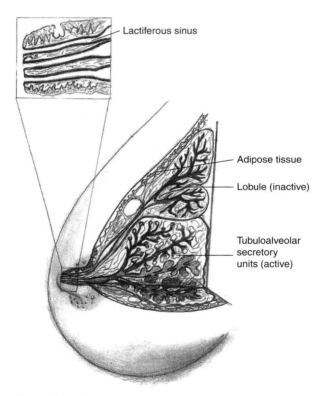

Figure 13.3   Mammary gland and nipple.

How is the mammary gland organized histologically?

Mammary glands contain compound tubuloalveolar glands with intervening adipose tissue divided into lobes by dense connective tissue.

What histologic changes occur in the breast during puberty and pregnancy?

Puberty: an increase in adipose and dense connective tissue of the breast

Pregnancy: ductal proliferation and differentiation

During the first half of pregnancy, the duct system differentiates with the appearance of many new alveoli. The gland secretes no milk. During the second half, there is enormous growth of glandular tissues and development is completed for the production of milk just before the end of gestation period.

How does the breast respond to hormonal changes throughout the menstrual cycle?

Follicular phase: Circulating estrogens cause mammary duct proliferation, while progestins released during the luteal phase induce lobular and alveolar growth in the breast.

Luteal phase: Growth often contributes to breast swelling, pain, and tenderness experienced before menses.

What happens to the breast after menopause?

The mammary gland undergoes reduction or involutes with the loss of estrogen. The secretory cells of the alveoli degenerate through apoptosis, and atrophic changes also occur within the connective tissue.

TESTES AND EXCRETORY DUCT SYSTEM

Surrounded by a collagenous capsule (tunica albuginea) with radiating septae, the testis is divided into multiple lobules. What structures are found in those lobules, and what is their function?

The lobules contain **seminiferous tubules** with simple columnar **Sertoli cells**, which assist spermatogenesis and maintain the blood-testis barrier. They also contain stratified germ cells at various stages of maturation undergoing spermatogenesis.

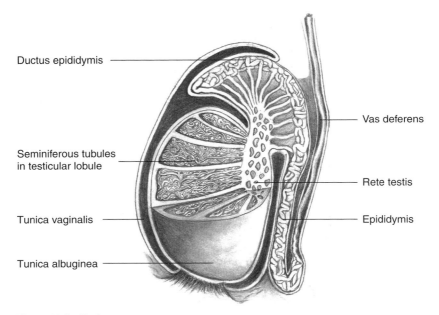

Figure 13.4 Testis.

Labels: Ductus epididymis, Seminiferous tubules in testicular lobule, Tunica vaginalis, Tunica albuginea, Vas deferens, Rete testis, Epididymis

What testicular and Sertoli cell structures contribute to the two layers of the blood-testis barrier?

Nonfenestrated capillaries contribute to the first level of the blood-testis barrier because they prevent the diffusion of plasma constituents into the testis. Tight junctions between neighboring Sertoli cells form the second layer of the blood-testis barrier. This border separates luminal contents from interstitial substances.

The development of antisperm antibodies often occurs when the vas deferens is cut and sealed during a vasectomy. The failure of what structure enables this phenomenon?

Failure of the **blood-testis barrier** affords interstitial immune cells unprecedented access to spermatocyte antigens. Consequently, antibodies are generated to these cellular and soluble antigens.

In addition to forming the blood-testis barrier and supporting germ cell maturation during spermatogenesis, what other functions do Sertoli cells serve?

See Table 13.1

Table 13.1 Hormones and Proteins Secreted by Sertoli Cells

Hormones and Proteins	Functions
Müllerian inhibiting substance	Stimulates regression of Müllerian duct structures in male fetal development
Androgen-binding protein (ABP)	Binds tubular fluid androgens and estrogens to maintain high, stable tubular fluid sex steroid levels
Inhibin	Inhibits pituitary follicle-stimulating hormone (FSH) release
Activin	Activates pituitary FSH release

At puberty, spermatogonia undergo androgen-independent maturation, proliferation, and meiosis until they reach the spermatid stage. During these stages, cytoplasmic bridges tie the cells together enabling symmetric maturation of germ cells at each stage. How do the germ cells differ from stage to stage during this androgen-independent maturation?

They differ in their **DNA content** (C) and **number of chromosome sets** (N). At puberty, type A spermatogonia mitose to produce several types A and B spermatogonia. Type B spermatogonia undergo mitosis to produce diploid primary spermatocytes (4C, 2N), which complete meiosis I to form haploid secondary spermatocytes (2C, 1N) and then haploid spermatids (1C, 1N) upon completion of meiosis II.

Spermatozoa originating in the germinal epithelium travel within what series of ducts on their way to the urethra?

Spermatozoa begin in the intratesticular ducts (seminiferous tubules, rete testis, and ductuli efferentes) and then traverse the excretory ducts (epididymis, vas deferens, ejaculatory duct, and urethra).

Epithelial cells from the rete testis through the epididymis contain abundant microvilli. What roles do those structures play in the maintenance of fertility?

Microvilli increase the surface area available for luminal fluid reabsorption and thus concentrate spermatozoa as they pass from the rete testis to the epididymis. Failure of this concentrating mechanism leads to semen more dilute than 40 million sperm cells/mL fluid and clinical infertility. Normal sperm counts in fertile men are greater than 100 million sperm cells/mL fluid.

In addition to concentrating spermatozoa, how does the epididymis function in spermatozoon maturation?

The epididymis activates a Ca^{2+} ion channel within the principal piece of the tail of the spermatozoon. This ion channel, CatSper, is important for forward motility.

Intratesticular ductuli efferentes have a ciliated epithelium atop a thick basement membrane and a circular layer of smooth muscle. How does this histologic organization affect fertility?

Beating epithelial cilia push immature, immotile spermatozoa toward the epididymis, where they will acquire motility. Similarly, circular smooth muscle contracts to propel the luminal fluid bolus toward the epididymis. Failure of those functions occurs in **Kartagener (immotile cilia) syndrome**, leading to male factor infertility.

How does its vascular arrangement permit the testes to maintain a temperature lower than the core body temperature?

Testicular arteries are surrounded by venous networks with opposite flow enabling countercurrent heat exchange. The testes are maintained at 32°C because of this heat exchange mechanism and their location outside of the pelvis in the scrotum.

Located in the testicular interstitium, Leydig cells contain abundant lipid vesicles. This microstructure indicates that Leydig cells produce fat-soluble hormones. What are the roles of Leydig and Sertoli cells according to the two-cell theory for spermatogenesis?

Stimulated by LH, Leydig cells produce testosterone, which diffuses into Sertoli cells found in the seminiferous tubules. Primed by testosterone and FSH, Sertoli cells assist spermatids with the final stages of maturation to spermatozoa, and they produce androgen-binding protein for high intraluminal testosterone maintenance. Sertoli cells also aromatize testosterone to estrogen for use in distal intratesticular ducts.

Ejaculation is a sympathetic reflex that can be divided into two parts—emission and ejaculation proper. Emission involves the movement of semen into the urethra via the vas deferens, while ejaculation involves propulsion of semen out of the urethra. What histologic structures found in the vas deferens facilitate its function in emission?

The vas deferens contains three thick layers of smooth muscle—inner and outer longitudinal layers and a middle circular layer. Reflex sympathetic stimulation of that muscle causes peristaltic contractions leading to propulsion of the bolus of semen into the urethra.

What are the three major accessory glands found along the ejaculatory system that supply fluid and preservatives to the seminal fluid?

1. **Bulbourethral (Cowper) glands**
2. **Seminal vesicles**
3. **Prostate**

Sixty percent of semen volume comes from the seminal vesicle, whereas 20% comes from the prostate. The bulbourethral glands supply the remainder.

PROSTATE

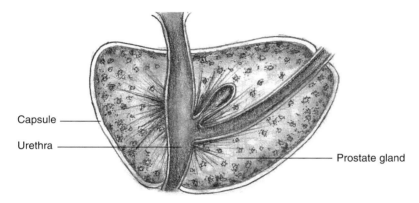

Capsule

Urethra

Prostate gland

Figure 13.5   Prostate.

The prostate is encapsulated and contains three zones: central, peripheral, and transition with a branched acinar secretory epithelium and intervening fibromuscular stroma. Based on this histologic organization, what is the function of the prostate?

An exocrine gland surrounding the urethra; its secretions contribute 20% of total semen volume. Containing cholesterol, phospholipids, fibrinolysin, and fibrinogenase, prostatic secretions liquefy coagulated semen.

Comprising 5% of the prostate, the transition zone is the glandular region immediately surrounding the prostatic urethra. How does prostatic glandular overgrowth and nodule formation or ductal obstruction lead to cyst formation in this zone? How do those processes manifest clinically?

Transition zone nodules and cysts compress the prostatic urethra causing a weak or intermittent urinary stream, incomplete voiding and leakage after urination, urinary frequency and urgency, and, in severe cases, urinary obstruction. Those lower urinary tract symptoms are associated with benign prostatic hypertrophy [(BPH), (hyperplasia)].

Comprising 70% of the prostate, the peripheral zone is the glandular region lying on the posterior prostate adjacent to the rectum. What two common pathologic processes occur in this zone?

1. More than 60% of **prostatic adenocarcinomas** originate from the peripheral zone. Prostate cancer may be detected through a careful rectal examination, with palpation of a hard, nodular prostate.
2. **Inflammation** may be detected by the presence of a warm, tender prostate.

PENIS

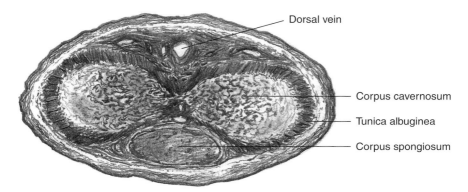

Figure 13.6   Penis.

How is the penis organized histologically?

Epidermis, dermis, subdermal smooth muscle (dartos), Buck's fibroelastic fascia, hyalinized tunica albuginea, two corpora cavernosa, and a corpus spongiosum

What two penile components are necessary for erection, and how do they function?

1. Corpora cavernosa
2. Buck's fascia

As the vascular erectile tissue fills with blood, venous outflow tracts are compressed against the tunica albuginea, which limits the degree of tissue expansion. In that way, the corpora cavernosa and Buck's fascia work together to create an erection.

What is the function of Buck's fascia?	It contains neurovasculature, encases the entire erectile complex, and forms a surface over which the skin slides during intercourse.
What is the clinical significance of Littré tubuloacinar mucous glands found in the penile urethra?	Their proximity to the corpus spongiosum facilitates the communication of infection into penile erectile tissue and nearby interstitium.

CLINICAL CORRELATES AND VIGNETTES

A 62 yo M c/o progressively decreasing force of his urinary stream, urinary urgency, and nocturia. Although he c/o decreased libido, his erections are adequate for intercourse. On digital rectal exam, focal nodules are palpated. An ultrasound-guided biopsy of the prostate reveals adenocarcinoma with a Gleason score of 7 out of 10. Which zone of the prostate is the adenocarcinoma most likely located?

Most adenocarcinomas arise from the **peripheral** zone. The Gleason grading system is based on architectural rather than histologic criteria. There are five grades; adding the grades for the primary and secondary patterns provides a Gleason score.

A 72 yo M c/o difficulty urinating. He reports he has difficulty initiating his urine stream, and after it begins, the flow is hard to maintain. He also c/o postvoid fullness and frequent UTIs. His digital rectal exam is unremarkable. His serum PSA is mildly elevated. What is his diagnosis and which zone of his prostate is hyperplastic?

Benign prostatic hyperplasia (BPH). The **central zone** of his prostate, surrounding the urethra, is hyperplastic. BPH is hormonally mediated; this zone has increased dihydrotestosterone (DHT) receptors on the prostate, resulting in hyperplasia. UTIs are a common complication secondary to urine stasis in the bladder. Treatment includes cholinergics to improve bladder contractility (ie, bethanechol), α-blockers to relax the bladder neck (ie, prazosin), or 5α-reductase inhibitors to prevent the formation of DHT (ie, finasteride).

A 36 yo F reports noticing a small lump on her left breast on a self-breast exam. She reports no pain, no skin discolorations, or nipple discharge. An ultrasound of the breast reveals a mass of heterogeneous echogenicity and irregular margins. The pathologic exam from a core biopsy reveals invasive ductal carcinoma. A fluorescence in situ hybridization is performed on the tissue to check for what markers?

Estrogen-receptor (ER) protein, progesterone-receptor (PR) protein, and human epidermal growth factor receptor type-2 (HER-2). ER and PR status have prognostic significance; tumors are less likely to occur when they are positive for ER and PR. By contrast, *erbB2* (HER-2/neu) overexpression indicates a worse prognosis.

A 24 yo F p/w intense abdominal/pelvic pain. She reports that this pelvic pain occurs every month at the start of her menses. She also c/o substantial pain during intercourse and unsuccessful attempts to become pregnant for the last year. On exam, there are palpable adnexal masses. On laparoscopic evaluation, there is uterosacral nodularity and ovarian cysts with large collections of old blood. What is her diagnosis and what is the other name for these findings?

Endometriosis. This occurs when endometrial tissue is found outside of the endometrial cavity. The described cysts are also called "**chocolate cysts.**" Common symptoms include dysmenorrhea, dyspareunia, abnormal bleeding, and a h/o infertility.

CHAPTER 14

Special Senses

PAIN, TEMPERATURE, TOUCH, VIBRATION, POSITION

Aδ and C fibers are associated with the transmission of which sensation?

Pain and temperature

Contrast the Aδ with C fibers:

See Table 14.1

Table 14.1 Characteristics of Aδ and C fibers

Fiber Type	System	Myelination	Speed	Termination Location
Aδ fibers	Glutamate-based system	Myelinated	Fast	Laminae I and V of the dorsal horn
C fibers	Substance P-based system	Unmyelinated	Slow	Laminae I and II of the dorsal horn

Describe the receptor mechanism of nociceptors and thermoreceptors.

Nociceptors and thermoreceptors have **free (or unencapsulated) nerve endings**. Containing receptors, like the vanilloid receptor-1 (VR-1) or vanilloid receptor–like 1 (VRL-1), these neurons respond to noxious chemical, proton, or temperature stimuli.

What are the four main types of mechanoreceptors?

See Figure 14.1
1. **Meissner corpuscles**
2. **Merkel cells**
3. **Pacinian corpuscles**
4. **Ruffini corpuscles**

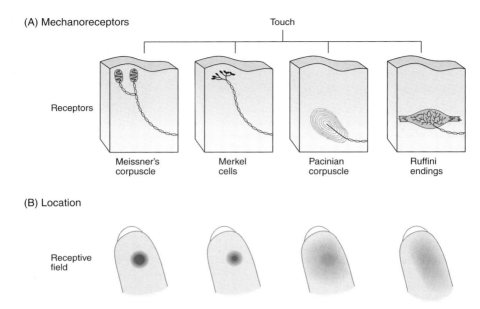

Figure 14.1   The four types of mechanoreceptors. (*Adapted, with permission, from Barrett KE, Barman SM, Boitano S, et al.* Ganong's Review of Medical Physiology. *23rd ed. New York, NY: McGraw-Hill; 2009.*)

Contrast the four main types of mechanoreceptors with their distinct functions.   See Table 14.2

Table 14.2 Characteristics of the Types of Mechanoreceptors

Mechanoreceptors	Location	Type of Sensation
Meissner corpuscles	Dermal papillae of glabrous (thick) skin	Fine discriminative texture and slow vibrations
Merkel discs	Basal epidermis	Light touch and sustained pressure
Pacinian corpuscles	Dermis, mesenteries, and periosteum	Deep pressure and fast vibration
Ruffini endings	Junction of dermis and subcutaneous tissue	Sustained pressure and skin stretch

What structures are involved in the transmission of proprioceptive information?

Awareness of the location of a body part in space likely depends on multiple sensory modalities present around a joint. The **integration of information from pacinian corpuscles, Golgi tendon organs**, and **muscle spindles** occurs in the cerebral cortex where a "picture" of the limb's location is formed.

MUSCLE LENGTH AND TENSION

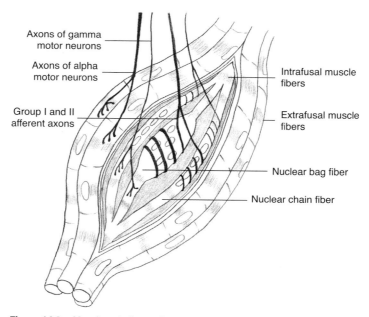

Axons of gamma motor neurons

Axons of alpha motor neurons

Group I and II afferent axons

Intrafusal muscle fibers

Extrafusal muscle fibers

Nuclear bag fiber

Nuclear chain fiber

Figure 14.2   Muscle spindle, nuclear bag, and nuclear chain fibers.

What are the three main receptors involved with muscle function?

1. **Muscle spindles**
2. **Gamma motor neurons**
3. **Golgi tendon organs**

Contrast the three different muscle sensory receptors.

See Table 14.3

Table 14.3 Characteristics of Muscle Sensory Receptors

Muscle Sensory Receptors	Location	Function
Muscle spindles	Between muscle fibers	Monitor the rate of change and maintenance of muscle length; also called nuclear bag or nuclear chain fibers
Gamma motor neurons	Ventral horn of the spinal cord	Modulate the sensitivity of muscle spindle input from alpha motor neurons; concomitantly activated with alpha motor neurons
Golgi tendon organs	Connected to muscle fibers at myotendinous junctions	Sense the level of muscle tension

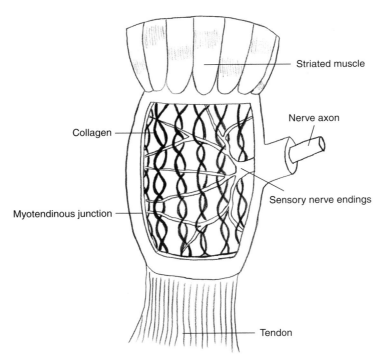

Figure 14.3   Golgi tendon organ.

TASTE AND SMELL

Of the different types of lingual papillae, fungiform, filiform, and circumvallate, which ones play a role in taste reception?

Fungiform papillae: located primarily on the anterior two-thirds of the tongue, receive facial nerve innervation

Circumvallate papillae: lie on the posterior one-third of the tongue, receive glossopharyngeal nerve innervation

The five taste modalities are sweet, sour, bitter, salt, and umami (a pleasant, sweet modality stimulated by monosodium glutamate that is distinct from traditional sweet). How do taste buds work?

Taste is a process whereby chemicals induce transmembrane receptor activation and modified epithelial cell depolarization to stimulate sensory neurons. Many compounds can trigger sweet and bitter receptors. A variety of **metabotropic G-protein–coupled receptors** depolarize these taste buds. NaCl activates epithelial sodium channels (ENaC) on salt receptors, protons activate ENaC and hydrogen cyanide (HCN) on sour receptors, and purine ribonucleotides activate metabotropic glutamate receptor on umami receptors to depolarize taste buds.

What are olfactory receptors, and how do they differ from taste receptors?

Olfactory receptors are **ciliated, bipolar neurons** that respond to chemical odorants and are directly **stimulated by specific chemicals**.

EAR

How is the external ear canal organized histologically?

Thin stratified squamous epithelium containing **hair follicles** with **sebaceous glands** and **ceruminous apocrine glands** with subjacent elastic cartilage

What is the clinical significance of the histologic organization of the outer ear?

Invasive resident or waterborne microbes (eg, pseudomonas) can easily traverse the extremely short distance between the surface and subchondral temporal bone.

What are the three layers of the tympanic membrane?

1. Keratinized stratified squamous epithelium (outer)
2. Vascularized, dense connective tissue bilayer (middle)
3. Simple cuboidal epithelium (inner)

What is the clinical relevance of the eustachian tube histology?

Dysfunctional cilia and seromucinous glands have a principal role in the development of middle ear inflammation and infections.

What is the relationship between the bony labyrinth and the otic capsule?

Otic capsule is the wall and the **bony labyrinth** is the **space** that **contains the membranous labyrinth**.

What are the components and their respective functions of the membranous labyrinth?

Cochlear duct, endolymphatic sac and duct, utricle, saccule, and semicircular ducts. The cochlea functions in hearing, the utricle (horizontal) and saccule (vertical) in sensing linear acceleration, and the semicircular ducts in rotational acceleration.

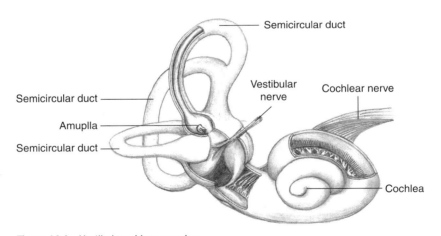

Figure 14.4   Vestibulocochlear complex.

How does the organization of the utricle and saccule relate to their functions?

The utricle and saccule sense **linear acceleration** or **head tilt (gravity)**. The sense organs within the saccule and utricle are called maculae. Both the saccular macula and utricular macula are **covered by a gelatinous mass,** called the **otolithic membrane containing concretions of calcium carbonate called otoconia or otoliths.** This loading of the cilia by inertial mass makes the organs sensitive to linear acceleration and changes of head position in the gravitational field.

COCHLEA

How is the snail-shaped cochlea organized?

Two and a half turns of the cochlear duct and the bony labyrinth forms three spaces: **scala vestibuli, scala media, and scala tympani**. With respect to the cochlear duct, the scala vestibuli lies superior, scala media within it, and scala tympani below it.

What four cochlear structures are associated with the development of clinical deafness?

1. **Spiral ganglion**
2. **Hair cells**
3. **Stria vascularis**
4. **Basilar membrane**

The spiral ganglion lies within the central cone of spongy bone about which the cochlear duct spirals and contains cell bodies of bipolar neurons that innervate cochlear hair cells. The stria vascularis and basilar membrane form the lateral wall and floor of the cochlear duct.

What effect do diuretics (eg, furosemide and ethacrynic acid) and anticancer agents (e.g., cisplatin) have on the cochlea?

Ototoxic drugs disrupt cells in the lateral wall of the cochlea, which maintain the low Na^+ and high K^+ content of endolymph, important for cochlear functioning.

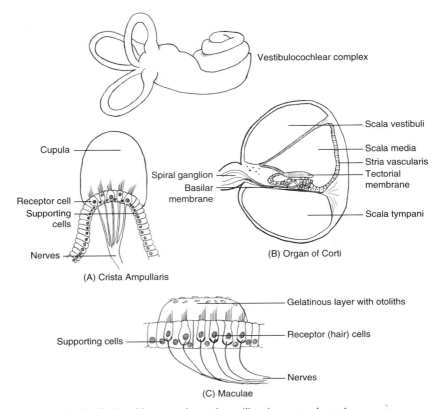

Figure 14.5   Vestibulocochlear complex and constituent sensory elements.

CLINICAL CORRELATES AND VIGNETTES

A 6 yo crying boy is brought to the ED for a progressively painful ear. His mother reports he had a low-grade fever and runny nose a week ago that is now resolving. On otoscopic exam, the tympanic membrane is red and bulging. What is his diagnosis?

Acute otitis media. His otoscopic exam is classic for a middle ear infection. Common organisms that cause a pediatric ear infection include; *Streptococcus pneumonia, Haemophilus influenza,* and *Moraxella catarrhalis.*

A 15 yo F c/o difficulty with hearing and a ringing in both ears. She reports her mother had a similar problem but only in one ear and had surgery for it. Her doctor notices hyperpigmented macules on her upper extremities. What is her diagnosis, and what type of hearing loss is this?

She has **neurofibromatosis 2**. The hallmark of this autosomal dominant disease is **b/l vestibular schwannomas**. One of the diagnostic criteria also includes a first-degree family member with a unilateral or b/l vestibular schwannoma. It is due to a mutation in the gene *merlin* on chromosome 22. The type of hearing loss is **sensorineural hearing loss**, which involves either the inner ear (cochlea) and vestibulocochlear nerve or central processing centers in the brain. By contrast, conductive hearing loss is due to the functional loss of the ear canal, tympanic membrane, middle ear, or its ossicles.

CHAPTER 15

Cell Membrane

LIPID MEMBRANE

Describe the fluid mosaic model of the plasma membrane.

The plasma membrane is a **semipermeable phospholipid bilayer**, in which integral components, such as lipids and membrane proteins, are free to diffuse laterally within the plane of one leaflet. Dynamic and deformable membranes are important for exocytosis, endocytosis, membrane trafficking, and membrane biogenesis.

What are the four main types of lipids that compose the lipid bilayer?

1. Glycerolphospholipids
2. Cholesterol
3. Glycolipids
4. Sphingolipids

What are glycolipids, and what are their functions?

Glycolipids are lipids with sugar groups. Found exclusively in the outer leaflet of the bilayer, they protect the membrane from harsh conditions by acting as a coat (eg, glycocalyx). These molecules are charged and function in cell-cell recognition.

What is the net charge on the cytosolic surface of the plasma membrane?

Negative charge. Phosphatidylethanolamine and phosphatidylserine, which are negatively charged due to their terminal primary amino group, are concentrated on the inner leaflet of the bilayer.

What increases and decreases the fluidity of the membrane?

Fluidity increases with increasing **temperature** and more **unsaturated double bonds**, creating kinks in the monolayer.

Fluidity decreases with an increase in the membrane's **cholesterol** content and **longer fatty acyl tails**.

What is the only type of molecule that is able to flip-flop between leaflets and is thus commonly found on both sides of the membranes of the lipid bilayer?

Cholesterol. Its small polar head group allows cholesterol to flip-flop between leaflets with limited energy expenditure.

Cholesterol has dual properties for the lipid bilayer. Name them.

1. Decreases membrane **fluidity**
2. Decreases membrane **permeability** to small water-soluble molecules

Note: it embeds its rigid steroid ring within the first few hydrocarbon groups of the phospholipid molecules, thereby further immobilizing the first few CH_2 groups of the hydrocarbon chain.

Cells are polarized. Name the side of the membrane that faces a lumen and connects to the outer body or a duct.

Apical region. A polarized cell is divided into regions, which have different compositions and functions. The basolateral region faces the capillary-containing tissue. The apical region faces ducts, has channels, and transports proteins embedded within it, which may alter the electrolyte concentrations of secretions.

Describe the asymmetry of the lipid bilayer.

1. Transmembrane proteins are often **glycosylated** only on the noncytoplasmic side, allowing for specific cell-cell recognition.
2. There is a net **negative charge** on the cytoplasmic side of the bilayer, resulting in an electrochemical gradient.
3. The cytosol is a **reducing environment**. Thus sulfhydryl groups, rather than disulfide bonds, form in the cytoplasmic side of the bilayer.

4. **Transmembrane proteins** confer functional asymmetry. Extracellular signals bind to the extracellular portion of a transmembrane protein, modify the intracellular portion, and generate a signaling cascade.

MEMBRANE PROTEINS AND LIPIDS

How are the two types of proteins associated with the cell membrane different?

1. **Peripheral proteins** are usually located on the cytoplasmic side of the inner leaflet and are bound covalently via a lipid group or noncovalently by interactions with transmembrane proteins.
2. **Transmembrane proteins** are amphipathic, meaning they have both hydrophilic and hydrophobic regions, and span the entire plasma membrane.

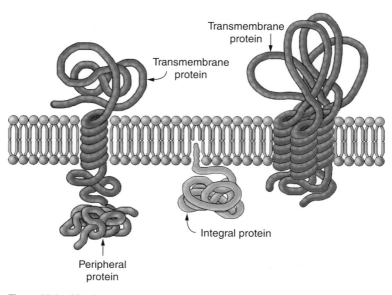

Figure 15.1   Membrane proteins.

What is the difference between a transmembrane and an integral protein?

Transmembrane proteins span the lipid bilayer and are thus functional on both sides of the bilayer. Integral proteins may have just a segment embedded in one of the leaflets with a lipid anchor.

What are the different ways transmembrane and integral proteins are passed through the membrane?

1. Single-pass proteins (α helix)
2. Multi-pass proteins (α helix or multiple β sheets in the form of a closed barrel)
3. Lipid-linked: thioester linkages
4. Carbohydrate-linked: glycosylphosphatidylinositol (GPI) anchor

How can the transmembrane segment of a protein be identified?

Transmembrane segments require 20 to 30 sequential **hydrophobic amino acids** and can be identified by a **hydropathy plot**.

Name some of the movements of the phospholipids within the membrane.

1. **Lateral diffusion** within the plane of a monolayer.
2. **Rotational diffusion** along the y-axis of the phospholipid.
3. **Flexion** of the hydrocarbon chain.
4. **Flip-flop** from leaflet to leaflet is rare and only occurs with the phospholipid translocase enzyme.

What type of solutions can extract the following types of membrane proteins?

1. **Transmembrane protein**
2. **Peripheral protein**

1. **Amphipathic detergents**: the hydrophobic ends of detergent molecules interact with hydrophobic segments of transmembrane proteins, thereby disrupting the bilayer and forming a water-soluble protein-lipid-detergent complex.
2. **Strong negatively charged ionic solvents**, such as sodium dodecyl sulfate (SDS) or buffers containing chelating agents, such as ethylene diamine tetra acetic acid (EDTA): changing the pH disrupts the electrostatic interactions and solubilizes the protein. Ionic detergents interact with and repel the hydrophobic polypeptide backbone, leaving the protein denatured and inactive. Chelating agents bind divalent cations, such as magnesium or calcium, which may form bridges.

Describe the erythrocyte cell membrane.

The membrane contains peripheral proteins **Ankyrin** and **Band 4.1**, which attach to the cytoskeleton by spectrin tetramers. The peripheral proteins associate with the transmembrane proteins, **Band 3** and **glycophorin**. Junctional complexes are points of attachment for spectrin tetramers.

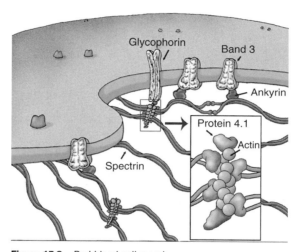

Figure 15.2 Red blood cell membrane.

The erythrocyte has only two transmembrane proteins. Name them.

1. Band 3
2. Glycophorin

The two transmembrane proteins of the erythrocyte cannot laterally diffuse. Why?

They are tethered by the cytoskeleton, allowing for the biconcave shape and flexibility.

Glycophorin is a much smaller protein than Band 3 but migrates similar to Band 3. Why does glycophorin run anomalously on an SDS gel?

Glycophorin is heavily **glycosylated** with O- and N-linked oligosaccharides and thus carries a heavy **negative charge**.

What is the key function of the Band 3 protein?

Band 3 functions as a **HCO_3^-—Cl^- anion exchange transporter**. It facilitates CO_2 excretion in the form of HCO_3^- by mediating the passive bidirectional exchange of HCO_3^- for Cl^- across the RBC membrane.

The free mobility of transmembrane proteins can be restricted. Give examples.

1. Interaction with the extracellular matrix or **cytoskeleton** (eg, Band 3 protein).
2. **Junctional complexes**: gap and tight junction proteins connect with the adjacent cell.
3. Formation of large **oligomeric arrays**: connexons are composed of six dumbbell-shaped polypeptide subunits that self-aggregate to form gap junctions.

CELL TRANSPORT

Name the three different types of cell transport processes.

1. **Passive transport**: moves a molecule down a concentration or electrochemical gradient across the lipid bilayer. No proteins are involved. It is also known as **simple diffusion**.
2. **Active transport**: energy requiring process transporting a molecule against a gradient.
3. **Facilitated transport**: uphill transport of a specific molecule is coupled to the downhill transport of another through protein channels. There is no energy source.

What is the difference between passive and facilitated transport?

1. **Specificity**: facilitated diffusion moves molecules through specific protein channels.
2. **Speed**: the maximum transport rate is limited by the number of transporters in facilitated diffusion. Also, the molecule does not need to enter the hydrophobic core of the lipid bilayer.

Name the properties of the molecules that can freely diffuse via passive transport.

Small uncharged nonpolar molecules such as O_2, CO_2, water, and urea can freely diffuse across a lipid bilayer.

Name the two main classes of membrane transport proteins.

1. **Carrier proteins** (carriers, permeases, or transporters): a specific solute binds, and the protein undergoes a conformational change to transfer the bound solute across the membrane. Transport through carrier proteins can be passive or active.
2. **Channel proteins**: they form aqueous pores that extend across the bilayer. Channel proteins transport solutes more quickly because there is less interaction between the solute and the protein. Transport is always passive.

What type of transport is the Na^+-K^+ pump?

It is an **active** transport process, involving antiport transport of three Na^+ extracellularly and two K^+ intracellularly. Phosphorylation is an essential characteristic of the pump, thereby placing it in the category of a primary (P)-type transport adenosine triphosphatase (ATPase).

What are the two primary functions of the Na^+-K^+ pump?

1. It **maintains constant cell volume** by decreasing the intracellular ion concentration, thereby decreasing the osmotic pressure.
2. It maintains a **potential difference across the plasma membrane**.

Many intracellular proteins function at an optimal pH. Describe three mechanisms/transporters that help maintain the cytosolic pH.

1. Na^+-H^+ exchanger
2. Na^+-driven Cl^--HCO_3^- exchanger
3. ATP-driven H^+ pumps

CLINICAL CORRELATES AND VIGNETTES

What is the osmotic fragility test?

This test measures the surface area: volume ratio of a cell and is a diagnostic test for **hereditary spherocytosis**. This test relies on osmosis, the passive diffusion of water molecules from a solution of higher water content to a solution of lower water content. As the surface area: volume ratio decreases, cells placed in hypotonic solutions lyse quicker. Hereditary spherocytosis leads to hemolytic anemia.

How do cardiac glycosides (digoxin, digitoxin) increase cardiac contractility?

They inhibit the Na^+-K^+ ATPase pump, which causes an increase in intracellular Na^+. This increases the activity of the Na^+-Ca^{2+} antiport, subsequently increasing intracellular Ca^{2+} and allowing for stronger heart muscle contractions.

How is human ABO blood group specificity determined?

Plasma membrane proteins are coated with glycoproteins or glycolipids. They confer individuality to each cell and facilitate cell recognition. The carbohydrate structure of membrane glycolipids and glycoproteins confers antigenic specificity. Human blood group A has a terminal N-acetylgalactosamine, B has a terminal galactose residue, and O has no sugar at that position.

How does insulin work in facilitating glucose uptake by the various tissues?

When insulin binds to its surface receptor on the membrane, glucose transport proteins (GLUTs) are translocated from the Golgi apparatus to the plasma membrane. GLUTs facilitate glucose uptake into the cells. GLUT 2 is located on the β cells of the pancreas, and GLUT 4 is located on muscle and fat cells.

The immune system discriminates self from nonself by polypeptide chains linked to a group of transmembrane proteins. What are these polypeptide chains called?

Histocompatibility antigens. These antigens, polypeptide chains, determine the individuality of the cell and help the body recognize self from foreign substances.

A 34 yo M c/o intermittent severe RUQ pain for 3 months. He reports N/V, and RUQ pain exacerbated by fatty, greasy foods. On exam, his RUQ is mildly tender, and he has splenomegaly. Labs reveal mild leukocytosis, normocytic anemia, decreased haptoglobin, and increased LDH. A RUQ US reveals stones in the gallbladder. (See Figure 15.3) What underlying disease increased his risk for gallstones, and what are the common molecular defects in this disease?

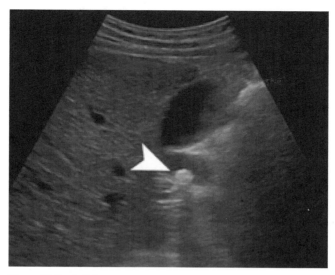

Figure 15.3   Gallstones.

Hereditary spherocytosis. Deficiency in the RBC membrane proteins (particularly **spectrin** or **ankyrin** proteins) leads to hemolytic anemia, commonly associated with splenomegaly, normocytic normochromic anemia, and pigment gallstones.

A 7 mo Caucasian boy p/w failure to thrive. Mother reports the baby is a poor feeder, passes greasy stools, and has had recurrent infections and pneumonia since birth. Birth history reveals meconium ileus. Physical exam reveals a malnourished infant with diffuse respiratory wheezes and rales and hepatomegaly. What is the first test you would perform to confirm the diagnosis?

A **sweat chloride test** revealing elevated concentrations of Na^+ and Cl^- three times the normal level confirms the diagnosis of **cystic fibrosis** (CF), an AR disorder affecting about 1:2000 children. The product of the cystic fibrosis transmembrane conductance regulator gene on chromosome 7 is a **chloride ion channel**. Mutations of this ion channel results in CF, and patients p/w malabsorption due to exocrine pancreatic insufficiency, recurrent bacterial respiratory infections, and increased salt loss in sweat.

CHAPTER 16

Cell Nucleus

NUCLEAR ENVELOPE

Describe the structure of the nuclear envelope.

It consists of a continuous outer and inner nuclear membrane with an intervening perinuclear space. The outer nuclear membrane is continuous with the rough endoplasmic reticulum (RER), which is studded with protein synthesizing ribosomes. The inner nuclear membrane contains proteins that bind to the nuclear lamina, a cytoskeletal structure juxtaposed to the membrane, providing shape and stability for the nuclear envelope.

What is the importance of the nuclear pore complex (NPC)?

The NPC is a **bidirectional "gateway"** between the nucleus and the cytosol or lumen of the ER for ions, messenger RNA (mRNA), transcription factors, ribosomes, histones, and other regulatory proteins.

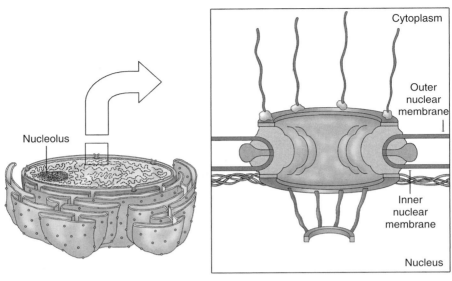

Figure 16.1   Nuclear pore.

What makes transport across the NPC unique as compared to protein translocation across other cellular membranes?

The NPC engages in both passive and active transport and allows macromolecules to pass in their fully folded conformation. This is in striking contrast with the extensive unfolding of macromolecules that is usually required for protein translocation.

How are proteins actively transported across nuclear pores into the nucleus?

Actively imported proteins have a **nuclear localization signal (NLS)**, a short 4 to 8 amino acid sequence rich in positively charged lysine and arginine. The NLS on the protein is recognized by cytosolic nuclear import receptors, which also recognize and bind the nucleoporins, a class of proteins, which make up the NPC. A similar process occurs for nuclear export into the cytosol, using nuclear export signals and receptors.

NUCLEOLUS

Describe the structure of the nucleolus.

The nucleolus is a **nonmembrane-bound** collection of ribosome precursors. It contains large loops of DNA, each containing a section of genes coding for ribosomal RNA (rRNA) and is known as the nucleolar organizer region.

What are the main functions of the nucleolus?

1. Ribosome synthesis
2. Transcription of ribosomal DNA by RNA polymerase I and III
3. rRNA packaging

What is the nucleolar size of a plasma B cell from a patient who has just been exposed to viral antigen?

Large—the size of the nucleolus is directly proportional to the cell's activity level. Cells producing a large amount of protein (e.g., immunoglobulin) require a large amount of ribosomal machinery.

CHROMOSOME ORGANIZATION

How are DNA molecules packaged into chromosomes?

1. **Histones** complex with DNA to form the basic unit of a chromosome, a **nucleosome**. Negatively charged DNA is wrapped twice around a positively charged octameric core of histone proteins. Each nucleosome is separated from its neighbor by linkage DNA, giving chromatin a **beads-on-a-string** appearance.
2. **Histone H1 protein** compacts the nucleosome organization bringing neighboring nucleosomes closer together to form the **30-nm chromatin fiber.**
3. This fiber supercoils and forms loops with the help of nonhistone DNA-binding proteins. This DNA-protein complex is known as **chromatin.**
4. Chromatin forms the higher order coils seen in **chromosomes**.

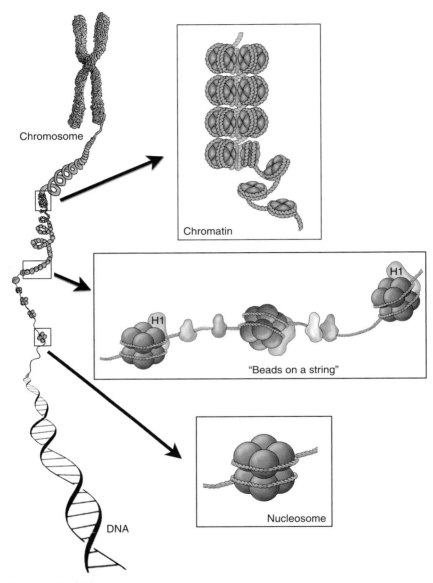

Figure 16.2   DNA.

Chromatin's structure is quite dynamic. Gene expression is dependent on decondensation of chromatin, which is regulated by two key mechanisms. What are they? Explain.

1. **ATP-dependent chromatin remodeling complexes**: these proteins are recruited to locally influence the chromatin and allow replication proteins to have access to the genes.

2. **Covalent modifications of the core-histone proteins' N-terminal tails**: Histones have tails that can be methylated, phosphorylated, or acetylated by histone acetyltransferases (HATs) and histone deacetylases (HDACs).

What other significance, besides reversibly altering the chromatin structure, do the covalent modifications have?

Stabilize the 30-nm chromatin fiber.

Different combinations of modifications attract specific proteins to a chromatin segment.

How are HATs involved in transcription?

Histones consist of a high proportion of positively charged amino acids, such as lysine and arginine, which effectively bind to negatively charged DNA sequences. Acetylation of the lysines neutralizes the charge thereby weakening the interaction between histone tails and DNA. This allows the chromatin structure to open up and **gives transcription factors access to DNA**.

What are heterochromatin and euchromatin? How do they differ?

See Table 16.1

Table 16.1   Heterochromatin Versus Euchromatin

Heterochromatin	Euchromatin
1. Transcriptionally inactive	1. Transcriptionally active
2. High degree of histone acetylation	2. Deacetylation
3. Highly condensed form of chromatin; packaged with histones and nonhistone proteins, which need to be dissociated from DNA for replication to proceed	3. Less condensed; loosely packed into 30-nm fibers and separated by adjacent heterochromatin by insulators
4. Located near centromeres and telomeres (areas of the chromosome with few genes)	4. Located near the nuclear pore complex
5. A typical cell in interphase will only have 10% of its chromatin in the heterochromatin form	5. The other 90% of chromatin is known as euchromatin
6. DNA replicated late in S phase	6. DNA replicated early in S phase

DNA SYNTHESIS AND REPLICATION

What does the semiconservative process of DNA replication mean?

The basic principle of DNA replication is that new DNA strands are formed by base pairing onto complementary DNA templates. The process is semiconservative because each daughter cell has a DNA double helix containing one old parent strand and one new daughter strand.

Name the different types of eukaryotic DNA polymerases and their key functions.

1. DNA polymerase δ: leading strand replication
2. DNA polymerase α: lagging strand replication and RNA primer synthesis
3. DNA polymerase β and ϵ: DNA repair
4. DNA polymerase γ: mitochondrial DNA replication

Why must there be a leading and lagging strand in DNA synthesis and replication?

DNA polymerase can only add a nucleotide to a free 3'-hydroxyl group. Thus, it only synthesizes DNA in the $5' \rightarrow 3'$ direction.

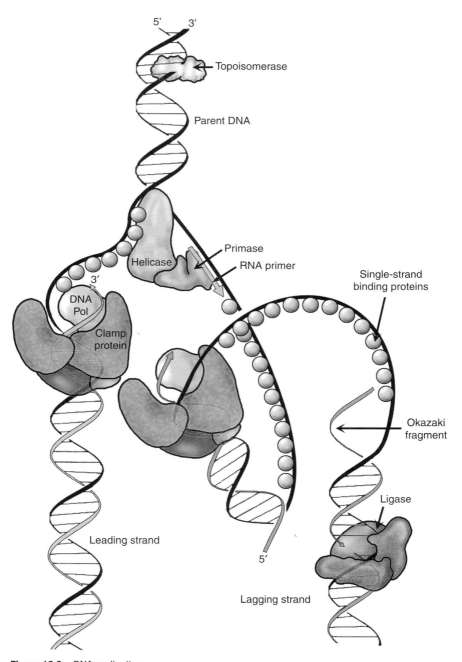

Figure 16.3 DNA replication.

How is the lagging strand synthesized?	The lagging strand is synthesized discontinuously by polymerizing short **Okazaki fragments** in the 5′→3′ direction.
Eukaryotic DNA replication involves six specialized mechanisms. Name the key enzymes involved and their functions.	See Table 16.2

Table 16.2　DNA Replication Enzymes

Steps	Enzymes Involved	Function
Initiation	Initiator proteins	Binds to the origin of replication to separate the two DNA strands; a replication fork is initiated.
Unwinding	DNA helicase	Separates the DNA double helix by creating a replication bubble with a replication fork that begins at each origin of replication.
	Single-strand DNA binding (SSB) proteins	Assist DNA helicases by binding to the exposed, single DNA strands to form stable, rigid, and straight DNA strands.
Untangling	DNA topoisomerase I and II	I: Provides a reversible single-strand break in the DNA to relieve stress in the twisted DNA helix and effectively form a swivel around the opposite, intact strand.
		II: Makes a transient double-strand break in the helix allowing the separation of two interlocked DNA helices.
Priming	DNA Primase	Synthesizes RNA primers along the lagging strand.
	DNA polymerase sliding clamp and loader accessory proteins	Prevents DNA polymerase from dissociating from the DNA template.

(Continued)

Table 16.2 DNA Replication Enzymes (*Continued*)

Steps	Enzymes Involved	Function
Unidirectional fork movement	DNA polymerase δ for the leading strand	Catalyzes the formation of a phosphodiester bond between the 3'-hydroxyl group of one sugar residue with the 5'-phosphate group of another nucleotide.
	DNA polymerase α and DNA ligase for the lagging strand	Synthesizes DNA fragments, known as Okazaki fragments.
Termination	Telomerase	At the end of a linear DNA sequence, there is no space for the RNA primer to sit and allow DNA polymerase to finish synthesis. Thus, a G-rich sequence, characteristic of the ends of DNA sequences, attracts the enzyme telomerase. Telomerase has an intrinsic RNA primer sequence and thus acts like a reverse transcriptase to synthesize terminal DNA sequences and to ensure complete replication. This is especially important for the lagging strand during DNA replication.

Describe the proofreading mechanism that is utilized in the DNA replication process.

DNA polymerase replicates DNA with very high fidelity using three key mechanisms.

1. It actively discriminates against mismatched bases by having a **higher affinity** for the correct nucleotide.
2. An intrinsic proofreading enzyme, **3'-5' exonuclease**, recognizes the insertion of a wrong deoxyribonucleotide base, excises it, and replaces it with the correct base.
3. **Strand-directed mismatched repair**: a mismatch repair complex scans the replicated DNA for mismatched nucleotides, removes a short segment of newly synthesized nucleotides, and replaces it with the correct sequence.

In strand-directed mismatched repair, how does the protein complex differentiate between the parental and newly synthesized DNA strands?

The template DNA strand is usually marked. In prokaryotes, a DNA methylase methylates specific nucleotide sequences. In eukaryotes, a single-strand break (nick) is created in the newly synthesized strand.

Name the four different types of DNA mutations.

1. Silent
2. Missense
3. Nonsense
4. Frame shift

DNA REPAIR

Compare and contrast the three major DNA repair mechanisms.

There are three major classes of DNA repair mechanisms:

1. Reversing base damage (direct repair)
2. Removal and replacement (excision repair)
3. Double-strand break repair (nonhomologous end-joining and homologous end-joining)

Describe three different types of DNA repair mechanisms.

See Table 16.3

Table 16.3 DNA Repair Mechanisms

DNA Repair Mechanisms	Steps	Types of Mutations Repaired	Special Enzymes or Comments
Base excision repair	1. Recognition 2. Cleavage (endonuclease) 3. Removal (DNA glycosylase and phosphodiesterase) 4. Replacement (DNA polymerase) 5. Ligation	Deamination, depurination (substitution or loss of nucleotide pair) mutations	DNA glycosylase, AP endonuclease, and phosphodiesterase
Nucleotide excision repair (NER)	1. Recognition 2. DNA unwound (helicase) 3. A patch of nucleotides removed (uvrABC) 4. Replacement (polymerase) 5. Ligation	Large, bulky changes in DNA double helix; a large sequence (patch) of 10-12 nucleotides is excised; eg, thymidine dimers	uvrABC enzyme, helicase, 7 XP repair enzymes; xeroderma pigmentosum is a cellular hypersensitivity to UV radiation due to mutations in any one of the enzymes involved in NER
DNA double-strand breaks	1. Nonhomologous end-joining: direct ligation of two DNA strands with complete breaks 2. Homologous end-joining: recombinant proteins and DNA replication proteins are used to repair the broken ends, using the intact homolgous chromosome as a template	Both strands of DNA are broken; often caused by ionizing radiation, oxidizing agents, replication errors	Advantage: may result in exchange of genetic information Disadvantage: risk of loss of heterozygosity or risk of translocations in direct joining (eg, Burkitt lymphoma, chronic myelogenous leukemia)

You suspect a disease called cell death is caused by defects in the DNA repair process. Describe what genes might be mutated and may be the underlying cause of this disease.

Any gene encoding a protein involved in DNA repair. Potential genes that may be mutated to cause cell death include:

1. AP endonuclease mutation prevents nicking of the defective deoxyribose sugar phosphate.
2. Phosphodiesterase mutation prevents excision of a defective deoxyribose sugar phosphate.
3. DNA polymerase mutation prevents both DNA replication and DNA proofreading.
4. DNA ligase mutation prevents the sealing of two DNA strands.
5. Uracil-DNA glycosidase mutation prevents recognition of cytosine that has been deaminated to uracil.
6. uvrABC enzyme mutation in this multienzyme complex prevents nucleotide excision repair of thymine dimers (eg, mutation in this gene and others involved in nucleotide excision repair can cause xeroderma pigmentosum).

Describe the mechanism of free radial injury.

Free radicals lead to cell membrane lipid peroxidation and ultimately DNA breakage.

How does the antibiotic class of fluoroquinolones cause bacterial cell death?

Fluoroquinolones directly inhibit topoisomerase II, also known as DNA gyrase. As a result, DNA becomes severely tangled during replication, causing cell death. Thus, fluoroquinolones are known as bactericidal antibiotic agents.

What is Bloom syndrome? What enzyme in the DNA replication process is mutated in Bloom syndrome?

Bloom syndrome is a rare autosomal recessive (AR) disorder that leads to an increased susceptibility to DNA damaging agents (eg, free radicals, radiation). The underlying genetic defect is a mutation in the enzyme **DNA helicase**. The clinical presentation includes immunodeficiency, dwarfism, spidery blood vessels in the skin (telangiectasias), photosensitivity, and increased risk of malignancy.

Name some common causes of free radical injury.

Radiation exposure, nitric oxide, and reperfusion injury.

Name some other syndromes resulting   See Table 16.4
from a defect in DNA repair.

Table 16.4 Syndromes With DNA Repair Defects

Syndrome	Gene Mutation	Phenotype
Hereditary nonpolyposis colorectal cancer	Mismatch repair enzymes (MSH)	Adenomatous polyps in the fourth or fifth decade of life leading to colon cancer
Werner syndrome	DNA helicase and 3'-5' exonuclease	Premature aging, cataracts, subcutaneous calcifications, muscle atrophy, increased risk of malignancy
Fanconi anemia	Heterogeneous; DNA cross-link repair process affected or mutations in proteins involved in forming a nuclear complex associated with DNA damage response mechanisms	Leads to bone marrow failure: anemia, leukopenia, thrombopenia, predisposition to leukemia
Cockayne syndrome	Mutations in genes involved in base excision repair	Light sensitivity, short stature, premature aging, no increased risk of cancer

CLINICAL CORRELATES AND VIGNETTES

A 13 yo M p/w fever, weight loss, anemia, and a localized area of pain in his right leg. He reports the pain is worse at night and aggravated by exercise. On physical exam, there is a localized area of swelling in the lower extremity near the knee. An x-ray reveals multilayered onion skinning in the diaphyseal-metaphyseal region. (See Figure 16.4.) Name the diagnosis and molecular basis for this diagnosis.

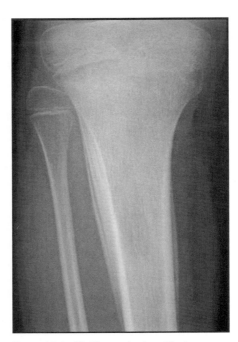

Figure 16.4   Multilayered onion skinning.

Ewing's sarcoma, due to a **chromosomal translocation of 11:22**, results in a chimeric fusion protein, which acts as a transcriptional activator, deregulating many genes associated with cell signalling, proliferation, apoptosis, tissue invasion, and metastasis.

A 4 yo M p/w severe sunburns and blistering over his face and arms. He has dry skin and photophobia. A mutation in what gene results in his genetic disease, and what malignancies are he at risk for?

Xeroderma pigmentosum is an AR disease resulting from defective excision repair genes, such as **uvrABC exonuclease,** leading to an inability to repair thymidine dimers. These DNA mutations typically form after exposure to UV light. The disease is associated with a risk for skin cancers, such as melanoma, at a young age.

Two of the proteins required for homologous end-joining recombination to repair double-strand breaks are encoded on the breast cancer genes-1 and 2 (*BRCA1* and *BRCA2*). What types of cancers do these predispose women to?

Breast and ovarian cancers

CHAPTER 17

Genes to Proteins

GENE ORGANIZATION

Why is the human genome so large?

The human genome contains both coding and noncoding regions. Coding regions are essential for polypeptide production and comprise 2% of the genome. The remainder comprises noncoding and transcriptional control sequences, which regulate protein synthesis.

Name some examples of the different types of noncoding regions.

Introns: intervening sequences in the primary RNA sequence that are spliced out; (introns are in the trash)

Gene families: for example, the globin gene contains embryonic, fetal, and adult subunits, all encoded on one gene

Pseudogenes: a gene that has been duplicated and is nonfunctional due to spontaneous mutations during evolution

Transcriptional control sequences and **RNA processing signal sequences**

GENE REGULATION

Many levels of gene regulation exist during transcription of messenger RNA (mRNA) and the subsequent translation to protein. Name the different regulatory points and give an example of each.

1. **Transcriptional control**: frequency of transcription is affected by the presence of enhancer sequences.
2. **RNA processing control**: genes that regulate alternative splicing can increase the variety of available proteins without increasing the number of genes in the genome.

3. **RNA transport**: RNA processing (eg, polyadenylation, 5′ capping) is required for nuclear mRNA export.
4. **mRNA degradation control**: RNA stability is regulated by sequences in unstable RNA and signal for rapid degradation.
5. **Translation control**: RNA editing alters the transcript before translation to produce different proteins from one transcript.
6. **Protein turnover control**: ubiquitin-dependent proteolysis affects the rate of short-lived and misfolded protein degradation.

What are the fundamental differences between prokaryotic and eukaryotic gene expression?

See Table 17.1

Table 17.1 Differences Between Prokaryotic and Eukaryotic Gene Expression

Prokaryotes	Eukaryotes
1. Transcription and translation occur simultaneously	1. Sequential process: mRNA is synthesized → processed → transported to cytoplasm → translated
2. Genes are contiguous sequences of transcribed DNA and lack intron sequences	2. Genes are often interrupted by intron sequences
3. mRNAs are polycistronic (one mRNA = several proteins)	3. mRNAs are monocistronic (one mRNA = one protein)
4. Only one RNA polymerase	4. Different RNA polymerases synthesize the different types of RNA RNA polymerase I: rRNA RNA polymerase II: mRNA, snRNPs RNA polymerase III: tRNA, rRNA
5. Utilizes an operon: one promoter regulates a cluster of contiguous genes, which encodes a set of proteins required to perform a coordinated function. This organization is called an operon	5. One promoter regulates one gene

What is the phenomenon of genomic imprinting?	A different phenotype is observed, depending on whether genetic material is inherited maternally or paternally.
What is the molecular mechanism of genomic imprinting?	The allele destined to be inactive undergoes cytosine **methylation** on **cytosine-phosphate-guanosine (CpG) dinucleotides**. The transcriptionally inactive gene is silenced by a high frequency of methylated CpG dinucleotides in the promoter regions, which block transcription factor binding. Only one allele is transcriptionally inactive, while the other allele, which is not methylated, is expressed.

TRANSCRIPTION (DNA → mRNA)

What happens when RNA polymerase II is added to purified eukaryotic DNA in a test tube?	Nothing; for eukaryotic transcription, addition of transcription factors is necessary. In contrast to bacteria, which only require RNA polymerase, transcription in eukaryotes requires additional transcription factors (TFIIs). Transcription initiation involves TFIID binding to the TATA sequence via the TATA-binding protein (TBP). TFIID binding distorts the DNA allowing RNA polymerase and other factors to bind and form the transcription-initiation complex.
What are the start and stop codons?	**AUG** is the mRNA initiation codon. It encodes methionine and N-formylmethionine in eukaryotes and prokaryotes, respectively. The start codon establishes the reading frame of the DNA sequence. Note: **UGA, UAA**, and **UAG** are the stop codons. (**U G**o **A**way, **U A**re **A**way, **U A**re **G**one)
Describe the two major differences between a promoter and an enhancer.	1. Location 2. Binding molecules

Table 17.2 Differences Between a Promoter and an Enhancer

Promoter	Enhancer
1. Located near the transcription initiation site usually close to and upstream of the gene it regulates.	1. Located close to or distant (either upstream or downstream) from the gene it regulates. May even be in an intron.
2. Binds RNA polymerase II and transcription factors.	2. Binds activators or repressors that influence the transcription-initiation complex.

List the similarities and differences between DNA and RNA polymerase.   See Table 17.3

Table 17.3 DNA Versus RNA Polymerase

Enzyme	DNA Polymerase	RNA Polymerase
Process	Replication	Transcription
Nucleotides	Deoxyribonucleotide triphosphates	Ribonucleotide triphosphates
Primer	Need RNA primer sequence	Primer not necessary to begin transcription
Region	Replication copies an entire helix	Transcription occurs in one specific region of one strand of the helix
	Only short sequences of the template are unwound until replication is complete	Sequence is unwound progressively as the RNA polymerase proceeds
Adenine paired with	Thymine	Uracil
Synthesis direction	$5' \rightarrow 3'$ direction	$5' \rightarrow 3'$ direction
Regulation	Highly regulated and occurs only during specific phases of cell cycle	Regulated by transcription factors
Accuracy	More accurate due to intrinsic 3'-5' exonuclease proofreading activity; error rate is 1 in 10^7 nucleotides	Less accurate; error rate is 1 in 10^4 nucleotides

What modifications must occur in order for the primary mRNA (pre-mRNA) transcript to be transported to the cytoplasm?

The pre-mRNA–protein complex is called the heterogeneous nuclear RNA (hnRNA). Processing the hnRNA involves three steps, which regulates translation and stabilizes the mRNA:

1. Addition of a 5' cap containing 7-methylguanine
2. Polyadenylation of the 3'-end (~ 200 adenine nucleotides)
3. Splicing introns out of the transcript. Only exons are transcribed; (**exons** are **ex**pressed)

What molecules are involved in splicing?

Spliceosomes, composed of several small nuclear ribonucleoprotein (snRNP) molecules, catalyze the splicing reaction.

What is alternative splicing?

A process by which one pre-mRNA sequence codes for many different proteins. There are two mechanisms for alternative splicing:

1. Trans-splicing involves combining exons from different RNA transcripts.
2. Different permutations of exons are created and combined.

You have isolated a protein that is similar in complementary DNA (cDNA) sequence to the transcription factor Bob. Although, Bob activates gene translation, this protein appears to repress it. The cDNA sequence of Bob is similar to your isolated protein, except for the lack of a short stretch of DNA sequences. Explain.

Alternative splicing can generate multiple transcription factor isoforms and has recently been discovered to be a mechanism for encoding transcriptional activators and repressors. By splicing out only the activation domain but keeping the binding domain sequence, a similar structural protein with a repressor effect is generated.

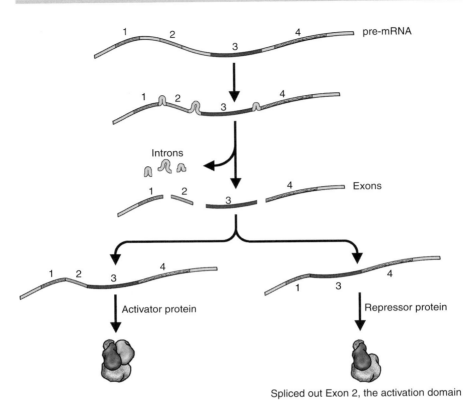

Figure 17.1   Alternative splicing.

TRANSLATION (mRNA → PROTEIN)

What is the function and structure of transfer RNA (tRNA)?

tRNA acts as an adaptor molecule between the amino acid and the mRNA template. tRNA is composed of 75 to 90 nucleotides in a cloverleaf structure. It has an anticodon, which complements the mRNA codon, and its 3′-end contains a covalently bound amino acid.

What is the function of aminoacyl-tRNA synthetase?

Charges the tRNA by catalyzing the addition of a specific amino acid to the 3′ terminal OH group of the tRNA. One ATP provides the required energy for peptide bond formation. Most cells have a different synthetase enzyme for each amino acid, adding to the accuracy of the process.

What is tRNA wobble?

tRNA molecules require accurate reading of only the first two positions of the mRNA codon and can tolerate a mismatch at the third position. tRNA wobble contributes to the **redundancy** of the genetic code.

The three steps of translation are initiation, elongation, and termination. Describe initiation in eukaryotes.

A group of proteins called eukaryotic initiation factors (eIFs) are key components in transcription initiation.

1. Initiator tRNA is recognized by eIF2.
2. The 5′ cap of the mRNA is recognized and bound by eIF4E, and the poly-A tail is associated with eIF4G. In eukaryotic initiation, both the 5′- and 3′-ends are important in recognition.
3. The small ribosomal subunit attaches to the 5′-end of the mRNA via recognition of the 5′ cap and its associated eIFs.
4. This complex is then brought to the small ribosomal subunit, which is itself associated with additional eIFs and the initiator methionyl tRNA.
5. The complex scans the mRNA along the 5′→3′ direction for the first AUG.
6. When a start codon is reached, all eIFs are released and the large ribosomal subunit binds to form the initiation complex.
7. Methionine is now positioned in the peptidyl (P) site.

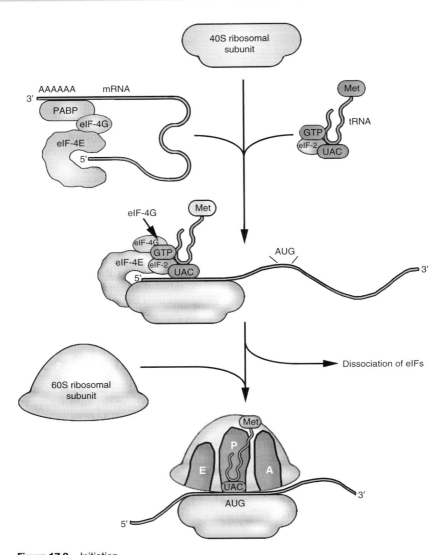

Figure 17.2 Initiation.

How does the prokaryotic and eukaryotic mechanism of initiation differ from each other?

Bacterial mRNAs lack the 5' caps and instead contain Shine-Dalgarno sequences, a ribosome-specific binding site. Bacterial mRNAs are polycistrionic, encoding several different proteins, which are translated from the same mRNA molecule. Thus, several Shine-Dalgarno sequences can be found on one mRNA.

Describe the steps of elongation and termination during protein translation.

1. Elongation occurs when the incoming AA-tRNA binds to the aminoacyl (A) site of the large ribosomal subunit. The initial methionine is positioned in the P site.
2. A peptide bond forms between the amino acids, and the methionine is transferred to the amino acid in the A site.
3. The ribosome then slides along the mRNA, and the uncharged tRNA enters the E site. An empty A site is now ready for the addition of the next amino acid.
4. Termination occurs when the ribosomal machinery encounters a stop codon, which is not recognized by tRNA.
5. Proteins known as release factors separate the polypeptide chain from the tRNA molecule.
6. The ribosome then releases the mRNA and dissociates into the large and small subunits.

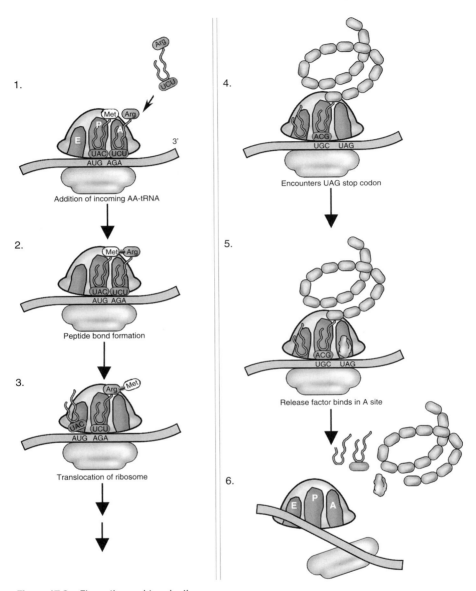

Figure 17.3   Elongation and termination.

Explain how release factors serve as an example of molecular mimicry.

In molecular mimicry, the structural properties of one macromolecule resemble or imitate those of another. Release factors structurally resemble tRNA molecules but lack a covalently bound amino acid. Consequently, they bind the A site of the ribosome and terminate translation.

Name several antimicrobial drugs which interfere with protein synthesis.

Antimicrobial agents often exploit the structural and functional differences between eukaryotes and prokaryotes to preferentially inhibit bacteria rather than host cells. See Table 17.4.

Table 17.4 Antimicrobial Drugs

Ribosome Inhibitors	Antimicrobial Drugs
30S ribosome inhibitors	Chloramphenicol, aminoglycosides (eg, streptomycin, gentamycin), and tetracyclines
50S ribosome inhibitors	Macrolides (eg, erythromycin) and lincosamides (eg, clindamycin)

CLINICAL CORRELATES AND VIGNETTES

Inheritance of both paternal copies of chromosome 15q results in what disease?

A deletion of the maternal copy of chromosome 15q leads to Angelman syndrome. This inheritance pattern is called uniparental disomy. Clinical manifestations include mental retardation, speech impairment, seizures, abnormal gait, and frequent inappropriate laughter. It is also known as happy puppet syndrome.

The mother of a 6 yo M is concerned about her son's tendency to overeat and his progressive obesity. She reports he has been exhibiting strange food-seeking behavior, including eating frozen food and rummaging through the garbage. On exam, he appears somnolent, is obese, and exhibits global developmental delay upon interaction. What do you expect to see upon genetic testing?

Prader-Willi syndrome is caused by a deletion of the paternal copy of chromosome 15q. Common clinical manifestations include hyperphagia, leading to obesity, mental retardation, and hypersomnolence.

A 40 yo M p/w jerky involuntary movements of his arms and face and progressive cognitive decline. This disease runs in his mother's family. What genetic disease are you concerned about, and what DNA mutation do you expect to see?

Huntington's disease (HD), an AD disease, commonly presents with chorea. Family history is a pertinent part of the patient's history. HD is one of the trinucleotide repeat disorders; $(CAG)_n$, which codes for glutamine, is repeated on the *HTT* gene on chromosome 4. It is categorized as a polyglutamine (polyQ) disease.

Name some other common trinucleotide repeat disorders and their repeated codon.

See Table 17.5

Table 17.5 Trinucleotide Repeat Disorders

Disease	Codon
Myotonic dystrophy	CTG
Fragile X syndrome	CGG
Friedreich's ataxia	GAA

A 53 yo M c/o chronic fatigue and abdominal discomfort. He admits to a significant loss of weight due to early satiety and has noted a decreased exercise tolerance. A peripheral blood smear reveals 150,000 cells/μL WBC count with a prominent basophilia and eosinophilia. What would cytogenetic testing reveal?

The presence of the **Philadelphia chromosome (t[9, 22])** is diagnostic for **CML**. The molecular event is a translocation of the *c-abl* protooncogene located on chromosome 9 onto a specific break point on chromosome 22, resulting in a **chimeric *bcr-abl* gene** with increased tyrosine kinase activity. In the early stages, CML presents with nonspecific symptoms such as fatigue and malaise. In the later stages, the patient presents with abdominal pain and early satiety due to massive splenomegaly. Treatment includes imatinib mesylate (Gleevec), which blocks the ATP binding site on the fusion protein and inhibits the tyrosine kinase.

A 32 yo M c/o bilateral flank pain and hematuria. He has a long-standing h/o HTN and renal failure. He also reports his father received a kidney transplant at the age of 26. A CT scan reveals multiple cysts in his kidneys bilaterally. (See Figure 17.4) What is the genetic mutation that runs in his family?

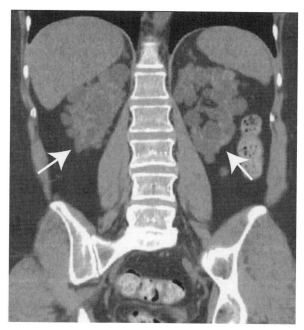

Figure 17.4   Multiple kidney cysts.

This patient has **autosomal-dominant polycystic kidney disease** (ADPKD). It is an AD disease with a mutation in the *AKPD2* **gene**. Patients p/w hematuria, urinary tract infections, and HTN. It is associated with polycystic liver disease, berry aneurysms, and mitral valve prolapse.

A 5 yo M was noted to become progressively weak by his concerned mother. The boy has difficulty rising from the ground, climbing stairs, and fatigued easily. On physical examination, his calves are disproportionately larger, and he walks with a waddling gait. Labs revealed an elevated serum creatine kinase. What is the diagnosis?

Duchenne's muscular dystrophy. It is an X-linked recessive disorder due to a deleted *dystrophin* gene, leading to accelerated muscle breakdown. Findings include pseudohypertrophy of the calf muscles (muscle replaced by fat), increased creatine phosphokinase (CPK), and weakness in the pelvic girdle area. The use of **Gower's maneuver** (See Figure 17.5), requiring assistance of the arms to "climb up" the legs to stand up, is characteristic.

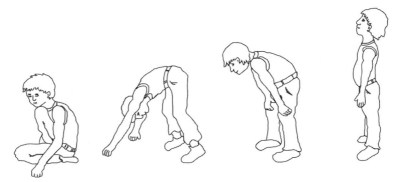

Figure 17.5   Gower maneuver.

CHAPTER 18

Molecular Biology Techniques

RECOMBINANT DNA

What are the key enzymes required to create recombinant DNA?

Restriction endonucleases and DNA ligase

What are restriction endonucleases?

Restriction endonucleases (**molecular scissors**) are bacterial enzymes that recognize and cleave distinct DNA sequence sites, which are often palindromic.

Describe the steps in creating recombinant DNA.

1. Using a specific restriction endonuclease, **cut** a large DNA molecule into several fragments.
2. **Separate** the DNA fragments by size using gel electrophoresis.
3. **Select** the DNA fragments that you wish to ligate or recombine.
4. **Recombine** the two fragments using DNA ligase.

Describe the process of gel electrophoresis.

Gel electrophoresis is used to **separate and obtain size estimates of nucleic acids or proteins.** It estimates unknown nucleic acid sizes by comparison with migrating fragments of known sizes. Applying an electric current across the gel causes the negatively charged nucleic acids to migrate toward the positive electrode. Smaller molecules move more readily through the matrix than larger molecules, thereby allowing for high-resolution separation.

DNA CLONING

Describe the two techniques used to produce DNA sequences in large quantities.

1. Selected DNA, recombined in a self-replicating genetic element (cloning vector), can be replicated in a host cell to produce many copies.
2. Polymerase chain reaction (PCR)

What is a cloning vector?

A **self-replicating genetic element**, (eg, a virus or plasmid) that carries a DNA fragment into a host cell (eg, bacteria or yeast cell). DNA fragments of 30 to 45 kilobases can be ligated into a plasmid vector.

Plasmid vectors are small circular molecules of double-stranded DNA that can self-replicate in bacteria. How are plasmid vectors used to clone DNA sequences? Describe the steps.

1. Using a restriction endonuclease, cut the plasmid into a linear double-stranded DNA molecule.
2. Cut the cellular DNA to be cloned with the same restriction enzyme.
3. Anneal the plasmid vector and cellular DNA fragment together via their cohesive ends to form recombinant DNA plasmids.
4. Covalently seal these recombinant DNA plasmids with DNA ligase.
5. Transfect bacterial cells with the recombinant plasmids.
6. As the cells grow, the recombinant plasmids also replicate to increase their copy number.

A complementary DNA (cDNA) library represents what part of the genome?

The part of the genome that is expressed is the **messenger RNA (mRNA)**. A cDNA sequence can be used to determine a protein's amino acid sequence, since it does not contain introns.

Describe the three major steps in a PCR.

1. **Denaturation (94°C)**: double-stranded DNA → single strand
2. **Annealing (54-65°C)**: two defined (forward and reverse) oligonucleotide primers hybridize to the complementary sequence of each strand
3. **Extension (72°C)**: the DNA polymerase adds deoxyribonucleotides and synthesizes the sequence of interest. This doubles your DNA.

Note: cycles of these three steps result in exponential amplification of the DNA sequence of interest.

What are the key biomolecular components involved in PCR?

1. **DNA** sample
2. Forward and reverse oligonucleotide **primers**, which flank the desired DNA sequence and are designed from the complementary strand.
3. **Deoxyribonucleotide triphosphates** (dNTP; A, T, C, G)
4. **Taq** (thermostable) **DNA polymerase**

PCR has size limitations—it is not the ideal technique for very large sequences. For example, patients with chronic myeloid leukemia (CML) may have a translocation mutation t(9; 22), which may be located within a large area of genomic DNA. For accurate diagnosis, what PCR variant could be used to detect and localize such a translocation?

RT-PCR (reverse transcriptase-PCR). By using mRNA rather than genomic DNA as the target sequence, cDNA is amplified using reverse transcriptase. Without the intron sequences, the sequence to be amplified is more manageable.

You are interested in cloning a gene that has yet to be cloned in your particular model organism. Describe how you would use PCR to clone this novel gene.

Sequences tend to be homologous among different species. For example, a high degree of homology exists between zebrafish and carp sequences. Primers designed from the carp gene could be used to clone the zebrafish gene of interest at lower annealing temperatures. This is called **degenerate PCR**.

DNA SEQUENCING

Describe the steps to the Sanger DNA sequencing technique.

Four separate reactions are run to sequence a single strand of DNA.

1. In each respective test tube, a DNA sample, DNA polymerase, a single primer, and four dNTPs are added to synthesize purified DNA.
2. A smaller amount of a single dideoxyribonucleotide triphosphate analog is also added to the mix.
3. The DNA primer binds single-stranded DNA, and a complementary sequence is synthesized until chain termination occurs with dideoxyribonucleotide incorporation.
4. These four reactions are gel electrophoresed, and the nucleotide sequence is read from the order of successive bands.

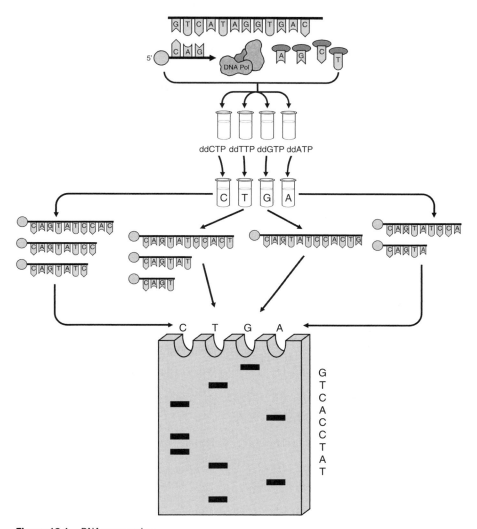

Figure 18.1   DNA sequencing.

Why do the dideoxyribonucleotides terminate chain extension?

The **absence of the 3′ hydroxyl group** on the incorporated dideoxyribonucleotide analogue terminates the growing DNA chain extension at specific bases.

The Human Genome Project (HGP) uses a different technique called the Shotgun sequencing technique to sequence DNA. Describe this technique.

For large-scale genome sequencing, the shotgun technique obtains many smaller overlapping pieces by randomly shearing the genome and assembling it into a complete sequence.

1. Randomly fragment the genomic DNA.
2. Construct a library by cloning the fragments into cloning vectors.
3. Sequence the fragments using universal primers for the vector.
4. Assemble overlapping sequences and reconstruct a large contig.

What are some applications for DNA sequencing?

1. Identifying mutations that lead to diseases or drug resistance.
2. Validating a cloning assay to ensure the accuracy of a cloned DNA sequence.
3. HGP goals include enabling rapid identification of candidate genes involved in specific diseases and identifying drug targets and disease mechanisms, especially in diseases involving chromosomal deletions.

BLOTTING ANALYSIS

Explain the basic steps to a blotting technique.

1. **Isolate** a cell-free mixture containing the protein or nucleic acid of interest.
2. **Fractionate** and **separate** by size, the biomolecule of interest using gel electrophoresis.
3. **Transfer** ("blot") the biomolecule of interest onto a suitable membrane.
4. **Hybridize** a labeled complementary probe to the membrane-bound biomolecule of interest.
5. **Detect** the biomolecule/probe hybrid by autoradiography

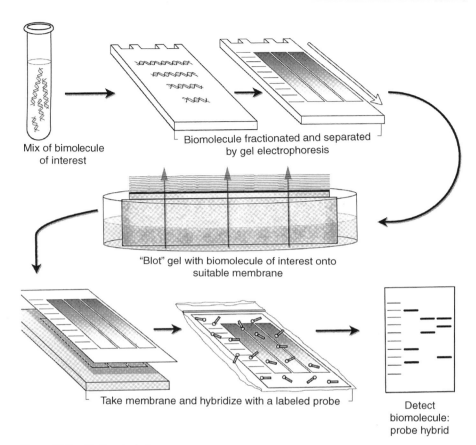

Mix of bimolecule of interest

Biomolecule fractionated and separated by gel electrophoresis

"Blot" gel with biomolecule of interest onto suitable membrane

Take membrane and hybridize with a labeled probe

Detect biomolecule: probe hybrid

Figure 18.2   Blotting technique.

What types of molecules are blotted for the respective types of blots:

Northern

Southern

Western

Northern blot: detects mRNA using an RNA probe

Southern blot: detects DNA using a DNA probe

Western blot: detects proteins using an antibody; also called immunoblotting

What are some applications for a Southern blot analysis?

1. Detects specific DNA sequences that are amplified, mutated, or deleted within mixtures of DNA
2. Studies the structure and location of genes by identifying restriction length polymorphisms (RFLPs)
3. Currently in use for the HGP to determine the order of the genes along chromosomes

What are some applications of Northern blot analysis?

1. Quantifies amount of mRNA present in sample. This is useful to detect and compare changes in mRNA abundance under different physiologic or experimental conditions.
2. Determines mRNA size.

What are some applications of Western blot analysis?

Western blotting detects antigenic determinants on protein molecules using antibodies.

1. Detects posttranslational modifications, such as phosphorylation or glycosylation.
2. HIV testing: acts as a confirmatory test for HIV

How would you find the binding site of a specific transcription factor on a DNA strand using a blotting method?

To detect specific DNA-binding proteins (eg, transcription factors), the initial step is to resolve the proteins of interest on a nondenaturing polyacrylamide gel. The separated proteins are then transferred to nitrocellulose and detected using a radiolabeled double-stranded DNA that contains the putative protein-binding site. The bound protein is then detected by autoradiography.

What does an enzyme-linked immunosorbent assay (ELISA) technique detect?

Antigen-antibody reactivity. Patient's serum is tested for the presence of an antigen (apply test-antibody to serum) or an antibody (apply test-antigen). The test-antibody or test-antigen is conjugated to a color-generating enzyme.

MICROARRAY ANALYSIS

What is the significance of a microarray experiment?

In a single experiment, an entire **gene expression pattern** rather than one specific gene, can be studied and monitored in response to a cellular event or to a specific growth factor, hormone, toxin, or different concentrations of the above mentioned. Some scientists use microarray experiments to do cluster analysis; for example, a group of proteins may be up- or downregulated in coordination secondary to a physiologic process.

Describe a microarray technique.

1. Extract RNA from the tissue or cell of interest.
2. Transcribe cDNA with fluorescent-labeled nucleotides from the extracted RNA.
3. Hybridize purified cDNA onto a DNA microarray slide, which has hundreds of different genes that serve as a probe for the purified cDNA of interest.
4. Microarray slides are scanned and images are analyzed based on signal intensity from the hybridized genes, which provide a measurement of the amount of bound cDNA.

What is the significance of microarrays and defining different types of leukemias?

Acute lymphoblastic leukemias and acute myeloid leukemias may appear similar in presentation. However, with microarray analysis, which distinguishes the different expression profiles, one can more accurately diagnose and prescribe the correct treatment, which is different for the different types of leukemias.

CLINICAL CORRELATES AND VIGNETTES

PCR has numerous clinical and research applications. What are these clinical applications? Give an example of each application.

1. **Detection of mutations in genetic disorder**: prenatal diagnosis of thalassemia and sickle cell anemia can be made by performing PCR on cells obtained by chorionic villus sampling.
2. **Detection of infectious agents**: hepatitis B virus may remain latent within chronically infected hepatocytes. PCR can detect viral DNA in asymptomatic patients.
3. **Forensic sciences, i.e.,** genetic fingerprinting: all individuals have a variable number of tandem repeats (VNTR) in their introns, or simple sequence tandem repeats (SSTRs or microsatellites). To identify paternity or a suspect in a case, a small DNA sample is used to amplify these unique sequences.

Name the tests used to (1) screen, (2) confirm, and (3) follow HIV infection, respectively.

1. **ELISA**: screening test, high sensitivity, rule out test; presence of antibodies (anti-HIV) produced by the patient is tested.
2. **Western blot**: confirmatory test, high specificity, rule in test; the presence of HIV proteins (gag, env, pol) is tested.
3. **RT-PCR**: viral load (RNA) is quantified; used to monitor a patient's progress by measuring the viral load during triple drug therapy.

A 28 yo African American F p/w her husband for genetic counselling. Her sister and husband's father suffer from sickle cell anemia. Because the couple is considering pregnancy, she is concerned about their future child's risk of inheriting this AR disease. They would like to determine whether she and her husband are carriers. What laboratory test is appropriate?

PCR and sequencing

A 45 yo M c/o dull, achy epigastric pain that improves after eating. He reports it is relieved by antacid medications. He has an extensive smoking history. You are concerned about peptic ulcer disease (PUD). What bacterium is most commonly associated with PUD, and what laboratory test can help detect this bacterium?

A sensitive test for *Helicobacter pylori* involves taking a stool or saliva sample and performing an *H. pylori* IgG **ELISA** to detect *H. pylori* antigens. Because *H. pylori* produces urease, a urea breath test is another rapid diagnostic procedure to identify *H. pylori* infections

CHAPTER 19

Organelles

MITOCHONDRIA

What is the main function of the mitochondria?

Energy (ATP) generation through carbohydrate and fatty acid metabolism via oxidative phosphorylation of ADP. Mitochondria are often called the **powerhouses** of the cell.

Where are the enzymes of the citric acid cycle and electron transport chain located within the mitochondria?

Citric acid cycle enzymes are located in the **mitochondrial matrix**, while **electron transport chain proteins** are found within the **inner mitochondrial membrane**.

What proteins does mtDNA encode?

Circular mitochondrial DNA (mtDNA) contains only exons, and it encodes **13 oxidative phosphorylation** and **electron transport protein subunits** and **2 ribosomal RNAs (rRNAs)** and **22 transfer RNAs (tRNAs)** for translation.

Despite mitochondrial ubiquity, why do mtDNA mutations result in clinical heterogeneity?

Each mitochondrion contains multiple copies of its unique circular genome. Thus, it is possible to have different copies, both wild-type and mutant mtDNA in each cell; this is called **heteroplasmy**. Also, a cell's mitochondrial endowment reflects its energy requirements. Nonuniform mitochondrial distribution and tissue heteroplasmy lead to the observed clinical heterogeneity.

Explain why mitochondrial cytopathies preferentially present as neuropathies and myopathies.

Tissues **high in energy demand** are more susceptible to mtDNA mutations. Common signs include muscle weakness, heart failure, exercise intolerance, dementia, seizures, droopy eyelids, and blindness.

Contrast the mitochondrial and nuclear genome.

See Table 19.1

Table 19.1 Mitochondrial Versus Nuclear Genome

	Mitochondria	Nucleus
Genome	Genomic circle; may contain multiple copies of the genome in the mitochondria	Linear molecule coiled into chromosomes; only two copies of the genome are in the nucleus
Organization	No introns	Both introns and exons
Genome length	Shorter (16,569 base pairs)	Longer (3.2 billion base pairs)
Inheritance	Maternal inheritance; egg contributes all of the mitochondria	Follows the law of independent assortment (an allele from each parent)
Mutation rate	10-12× higher than nuclear DNA	Low; many proofreading mechanisms

Explain the concept of chemiosmotic coupling in ATP synthesis.

Protein complexes in the inner mitochondrial membrane generate ATP from an electrochemical proton gradient. As electrons are transferred through a series of electron carrier complexes, it generates energy to pump protons against their concentration gradient to the intermembrane space. This electrochemical gradient is harnessed to generate ATP by allowing the protons to flow "downhill" through an ATP synthase protein. See Figure 19.1.

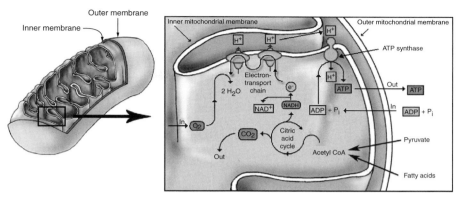

Figure 19.1   Mitochondria.

What is the significance of the mitochondrial cristae?

The inner mitochondrial membrane is folded into cristae, creating a **greater surface area** for incorporating proteins involved in the synthesis of ATP, thereby **maximizing oxidative metabolism**.

How and why do the inner and outer mitochondrial membranes differ in permeability?

The outer membrane contains **porins**, or channels, which allow transport of small molecules into the intermembrane space. The inner membrane is impermeable to ions, which creates the potential energy and electrochemical gradient required for ATP synthesis.

Your protein of interest (YPI) is a protein encoded by the nuclear genome and is located in the mitochondrial matrix. Explain how this protein arrives in the matrix after protein translation.

Cytosol: YPI translation yields a protein containing an amino terminal mitochondrial localizing sequence (MLS), which allows posttranslational sorting to the outer mitochondrial surface. Heat shock proteins (eg, Hsp70) act as chaperones to hold cytosolic YPI in an unfolded state.

Outer mitochondrial membrane: YPI is transferred across the outer mitochondrial membrane into the intermembrane space through a protein translocator, the Tom complex (translocase of the outer mitochondrial membrane).

Inner mitochondrial membrane: YPI is imported through the Tim complex (translocase of the inner mitochondrial membrane) and remains in the matrix where the MLS sequence is cleaved.

What cell in the body lacks mitochondria?	**RBCs.** RBCs depend solely on glycolysis, and mutations in any of the glycolytic enzymes (eg, hexokinase, aldolase, pyruvate kinase) result in hemolytic anemia.
What happens in cyanide poisoning?	Cyanide **inactivates cytochrome oxidase** (cytochrome aa3), which is involved in the **mitochondrial electron transport chain**. By interfering with cellular respiration, tissues with high O_2 requirement are affected first (eg, brain, heart, liver). A common finding is the smell of bitter almonds on the breath. The antidote is sodium nitrite.

ENDOPLASMIC RETICULUM

The endoplasmic reticulum (ER) is classically divided into the smooth (SER) and rough (RER) regions by morphology. What are the distinguishing features of each?	See Table 19.2

Table 19.2 Rough Endoplasmic Reticulum Versus Smooth Endoplasmic Reticulum

Rough ER	Smooth ER
1. **Granular** appearance due to the abundance of bound ribosomes	1. Appears **smooth** due to the lack of bound ribosomes
2. Primary site of **secretory protein synthesis**	2. Primary site for **lipid biosynthesis**, **steroid hormone synthesis**, **intracellular calcium storage** (in muscle cells, also known as sarcoplasmic reticulum), and **detoxification** of dangerous metabolites via the cytochrome p450 enzymes

State whether each of the following tissues would be enriched in RER or SER and for which unique metabolic function this specification is useful:

Hepatocytes of an epileptic (treated with barbiturates)	The hepatocyte's ability to break down toxic small molecules (eg, barbiturates) is due to the demethylases and oxidases indigenous to the **SER**.
Cardiomyocytes	The heart's ability to respond to electrical stimuli relies on efficient Ca^{2+} ion storage in and release from the sarcoplasmic reticulum. The sarcoplasmic reticulum is actually **SER** optimized for this specific task.
Adrenal gland, zona fasciculata	Many enzymes required for steroid hormone biosynthesis reside in the **SER**.
Plasma cell	Plasma cells, which synthesize and secrete antibodies, are enriched in **RER** because of the abundance of ribosomes attempting to translocate their nascent immunoglobulin chains into the RER and the secretory pathway.

Describe the steps involved in creating an integral membrane protein.

1. During translation, when the nascent signal sequence emerges from the ribosome, the signal recognition particle (SRP) recognizes and binds it.
2. The SRP brings the mRNA-ribosome complex to the ER membrane, and it binds to the SRP receptor, which temporarily ceases translation.
3. As the SRP is released, the ribosome binds to the Sec 61 protein complex, a membrane translocation protein.
4. The signal sequence is inserted into a membrane channel.
5. Translation resumes and the growing polypeptide chain is translocated across the membrane.
6. Cleavage of the signal sequence by signal peptidase releases the polypeptide into the lumen of the ER.

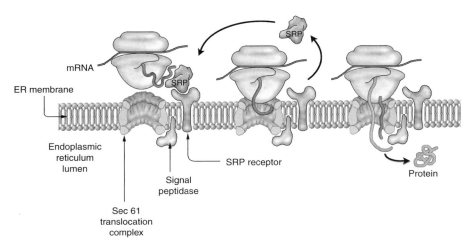

Figure 19.2   Protein translocation.

A G-protein–coupled photoreceptor in the retina has seven transmembrane segments. Its N-terminus is exposed to the extracellular environment while its C-terminus is maintained within the cell for signal transduction. How should this receptor be oriented in the ER and in a transport vesicle to ensure that it is properly delivered to the cell surface?

The lumen of both the ER and any vesicle is topologically equivalent to the extracellular space. The N-terminus of this G-protein must therefore be luminal. Ultimately, the C-terminus of this receptor will be cytoplasmic, and it will maintain contact with the cytoplasm both in the ER membrane and as it travels to the cell surface.

Despite very diverse activities within the ER, protein disulfide isomerase (catalyzes formation and breakage of disulfide bonds), BiP (chaperone protein), and many glycosyl transferases (glycosylating proteins) all share a common C-terminal sequence. Why?

Retention in the ER. Most ER proteins exist to assist in and maintain quality control over the protein folding/assembly process. Soluble and some ER membrane proteins possess the C-terminal sequence KDEL, which concentrates these proteins by returning them via retrograde transport whenever they are inadvertently admitted to the secretory pathway. Other membrane proteins possess the C-terminal KKXX consensus for the same purpose.

Describe the unfolded protein response (UPR).	Metabolic challenges such as starvation, misfolded protein accumulation, or exposure to extreme redox environments require a compensatory upregulation of ER activity for survival. The UPR is a transcriptional and translational response to this ER stress. Responses include stalled translocation of new proteins into the ER and upregulation of resident ER chaperones. Apoptotic pathways are induced if the UPR cannot overcome chronic ER stress.

GOLGI COMPLEX

What are the basic functions of the Golgi apparatus?	1. **Sorts** ER proteins and dispatches them to the plasma membrane, secretory granules, or to lysosomes from the trans Golgi network. 2. **Carbohydrate factory.** Adds O-linked oligosaccharides to serine and threonine residues and modifies N-linked oligosaccharides. 3. Attaches **mannose-6-phosphate (M6P) tags** to lysosomal proteins. 4. **Proteoglycan modifications** (eg, O-linked glycosylation and sulfation of tryosoines).
What is the structure of the Golgi apparatus?	The Golgi apparatus consists of stacks of four to six flattened cisternae. Golgi vesicles transport proteins and lipids between the cisternae, as well as to and from the Golgi apparatus itself. Golgi stacks have a cis and a trans face, which act as sorting stations that connect to the cisternae. Proteins and lipids from the ER enter the Golgi at the cis Golgi network and exit from the trans Golgi network. Vesicles may also return to the ER via the cis Golgi network.

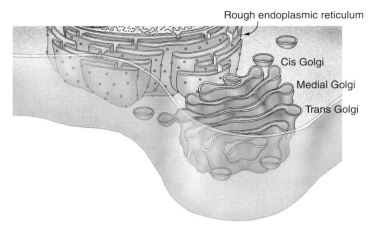

Figure 19.3   Golgi apparatus.

How are Golgi cisternae like a factory assembly line?

Each cisterna has its own enzyme system that functions in the oligosaccharide processing pathway as the protein moves successively through the cis, medial, and trans cisternae. In this way, they resemble a factory assembly line.

What membrane-associated enzymatic reactions occur in the Golgi networks and cisternal compartments?

See Table 19.3

Table 19.3   Golgi Compartments and Their Function

Location	Enzymatic Reactions
Cis Golgi network	Phosphorylation of oligosaccharides on proteins destined for the lysosome.
Cis cisterna	High mannose chains are trimmed to M5 by mannosidase I.
Medial cisterna	Mannose removal, GlcNAc attachment by GlcNAc transferase I, and O-linked glycosylation (sugars added to the hydroxyl groups of selected serines and threonines side chains) occur here.
Trans cisterna	Terminal sugars (galactosyl residues) and sialic acid (NANA) are added. Addition of NANA gives proteins a high negative charge.
Trans Golgi network	Tyrosines are sulfated. It also has same functions as the trans cisterna.

Describe the two models explaining the transport between the Golgi compartments.

1. The **cisternal maturation model** supports the theory that Golgi compartments are dynamic structures that gain and lose enzymatic functions as they carry proteins from the cis to the trans cisterna. Recent research supports this model with evidence that compartment maturation exists, and the rate of protein transport is similar to that of maturation of the compartments.
2. **Vesicular transport model.** In this model, transport vesicles ship proteins between the Golgi cisternae to each compartment with stable, resident enzymes and proteins.

If a glycosylated molecule is attached to the luminal side of the Golgi membrane, which side of the cellular plasma membrane will it face after the transport?

The molecule will face the extracellular side of the plasma membrane. This is because the Golgi, ER, and transport vesicle lumens are equivalent to the cell's extracellular space. This constraint results in plasma membrane asymmetry where more carbohydrates face the extracellular rather than intracellular space.

Which types of cells have a prominent Golgi network?

Specialized secretory cells have prominent Golgi networks. Intestinal goblet cells have large vesicles that exit the trans Golgi network and travel to the plasma membrane for secretion. In this way, polysaccharide-rich mucus is secreted into the intestinal lumen. Other cell types with prominent Golgi networks include pancreatic acinar cells, plasma cells, neurons releasing neurotransmitters, and endocrine cells.

If the forward pathway of transport from the ER to the Golgi is disrupted, what will happen to the lipids and proteins residing within the Golgi?

Transport from the ER to the Golgi is mediated by transport vesicles, while the return pathway from the Golgi to the ER is mediated by microtubule-based membrane tubes. Brefeldin A disrupts the forward pathway from the ER to the Golgi by interrupting coat assembly needed for transport vesicle budding. However, microtubules and membrane tubes are not affected, so backward transport (Golgi → ER) remains intact. As a result of brefeldin A, Golgi proteins and lipids will cycle back to the ER.

What are the three major destinations of proteins leaving the trans Golgi network?

1. **Lysosomes**: proteins going to lysosomes are tagged with M6P markers.
2. **Secretory vesicles**: proteins with specific sorting signals are transferred to secretory vesicles in specialized secretory cells.
3. **Plasma membrane**: the nonselective default pathway in unpolarized cells automatically transports proteins without specific signals to the cell surface. Polarized cells use more specific signals in order to direct proteins to the apical or the basolateral surface.

LYSOSOMES

What is the main function of lysosomes?

Lysosomes are the garbage disposal system of the cell. This organelle contains **hydrolytic enzymes** that digest selected macromolecules. The lysosomal membrane also forms a barrier to contain the enzymes within the organelle. Once digestion of the macromolecules is complete, by-products are transported to the cytosol to be recycled or removed by the cell.

What are some of the unique features of the lysosomal membrane?

Lysosomal membranes contain **H⁺ pumps** powered by ATP to maintain the luminal acidic pH of 5. If these enzymes leak out of the lysosome, they will not function at the cell's pH of 7.2. Membrane proteins are also heavily glycosylated in order to protect them from these lysosomal proteases.

How are materials delivered to lysosomes?

1. Digestive enzymes from the ER are transported to lysosomes via the **Golgi network**.
2. Macromolecules can be endocytosed into early **endosomes**, which eventually fuse to become late endosomes. As the pH becomes more acidic, the late endosomes transform into mature lysosomes.
3. Microorganisms and other macromolecules may be phagocytosed to form **phagosomes**.
4. **Autophagy** is the disposal system for obsolete cellular organelles. Membranes surround and enclose organelles targeted for destruction and form autophagosomes. These then fuse with late endosomes or lysosomes.

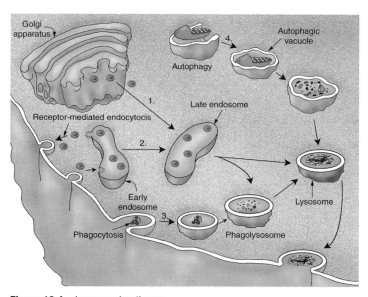

Figure 19.4   Lysosomal pathway.

How does the early endosome act as a sorting station?

If a receptor releases its ligand and changes its structural shape in the early endosome, the ligands are then degraded by the lysosome. The receptor may be transported to lysosomes for destruction (eg, epidermal growth factor (EGF) receptor) or may return to their original site in the lipid membrane (eg, low-density lipoprotein (LDL) receptor).

What special marker is used to identify and sort lysosomal hydrolases within the Golgi?

Mannose 6-phosphate (M6P) is a tag that attaches to N-linked oligosaccharides on modified lysosomal enzymes in the cis Golgi network. M6P receptors are found in the trans Golgi network, where they attach to lysosomal hydrolases and package them into transport vesicles destined for fusion with late endosomes.

What is the scavenger pathway for lysosomal hydrolases?

M6P receptors are sent to the plasma membrane of the cell to recapture the enzymes and return them to the lysosomes. Receptor-mediated endocytosis is used to return the escaped enzymes to early, then late endosomes, which eventually form lysosomes.

How does the Golgi apparatus add M6Ps to lysosomal hydrolases?

The Golgi uses two enzymes to catalyze this reaction in the cis Golgi network.

1. **GlcNAc-phosphotransferase**: it attaches a GlcNAc-phosphate to the sixth position of some mannose residues on N-linked oligosaccharides.
2. **GlcNAc-phosphoglycosidase**: it cleaves off GlcNAc residues to expose M6P residues. The more M6P residues added to the oligosaccharides, the greater its affinity for the M6P receptor.

| If there is a defective or missing GlcNAc phosphotransferase, how will that affect the lysosomal hydrolase sorting process? | Lysosomal hydrolases will not be sorted and will be transported through the default pathway for secretion. This results in buildup of undigested materials within the lysosome, which forms inclusions. This results in a lysosomal storage disease called **I-cell disease** (inclusion-cell disease), characterized by course facial features, gingival hypertrophy, and joint stiffness. |
| Name some common lysosomal storage diseases and their missing lysosomal enzyme. | See Table 19.4 |

Table 19.4 Lysosomal Storage Diseases

Lysosomal Storage Disorders	Enzyme
Tay-Sachs disease	Hexosaminidase A
Gaucher disease	β-Glucocerebrosidase
Niemann-Pick disease	Sphingomyelinase
Pompe disease	α-1,4-glucosidase
Fabry disease	α-Galactosidase A
Krabbe disease	Galactocerebrosidase
Metachromatic leukodystrophy	Arylsulfatase A

CLINICAL CORRELATES AND VIGNETTES

A 30 yo M undergoes general anesthesia for surgery. Suddenly his muscles become rigid; he becomes tachycardic, tachypneic, and febrile. What is the mechanism of the intravenous drug that will reverse his condition and save his life?

Malignant hyperthermia is an AD metabolic myopathy caused by an abnormal release of calcium from the SR of skeletal myocytes and an ineffective reuptake afterward. **Dantrolene** prevents the release of Ca^{2+} from the SR and must be given immediately. Life-threatening malignant hyperthermia is characterized by acute fever, tachypnea, tachycardia, and rigidity. It is often precipitated by anesthetics (eg, halothane) or muscle relaxants (eg, succinylcholine).

An Ashkenazi Jewish family brings in their 4 mo infant with progressive hypotonia, hyperreflexia, deteriorating motor skills, and macular cherry red spots on ophthalmic examination. The patient appears to have an enlarged head. The infant goes on to develop seizures and blindness, dying by the age of 3 years. What enzyme is absent or deficient in this patient's cells?

Tay-Sachs disease is defective in hexosaminidase A leading to an accumulation of GM2 gangliosides within lysosomes. This illness commonly affects the Ashkenazi Jewish population with a carrier rate estimated to be about 1:30. Patients with Tay-Sachs typically have normal motor development for the first 2 to 6 months, and then their condition progressively deteriorates.

A 3 yo child dies of a neurodegenerative disease. Tissues taken from the liver, spleen, lymph nodes, and skin are prepared and examined under a microscope. The samples reveal foamy histiocytes filled with sphingomyelin and cholesterol. What rare AR disease did this patient succumb to?

This patient had Niemann-Pick disease, which is a lipid storage disorder due to a deficiency of sphingomyelinase. Intracellular accumulations of sphingomyelin that lead to foam cell production are pathognomonic for this disease. Other common features of this illness include hepatosplenomegaly, neurologic degeneration, anemia, fever, and a cherry red spot seen on ophthalmic examination.

A 4 mo F infant presents to her pediatrician with macroglossia, an enlarged heart, and progressive hypotonia. The patient has failure to thrive due to difficulties with feeding and respiration. She is found to have a defect in α-glucosidase, which has led to an accumulation of glycogen within the lysosomes. What type of lysosomal storage disease does this patient have?

This patient has glycogen storage disease type II, called Pompe disease. It is inherited in an AR pattern. The defective α-glucosidase is a lysosomal enzyme used to break down glycogen. As a result, glycogen accumulates within lysosomes. Cardiorespiratory failure before the age of 2 years is often the cause of death for these patients.

Relief workers identify a famine survivor with extensive bruising on the skin, swollen and bleeding gums, missing teeth, and anemia. Mass spectrometric analysis reveals that tropocollagen peptides are slightly smaller than usual. What is the diagnosis?

Scurvy. Vitamin C is a required cofactor for the hydroxylation of procollagen proline and lysine residues in the RER. This hydroxylation step is required for the subsequent cross-linking of adjacent tropocollagen chains by lysyl oxidase. The result is extremely weak collagen fibrils, and a pathological state that can be reversed by dietary modification and vitamin C supplementation.

How do animals use brown adipose tissue mitochondria to generate heat?

Brown adipose tissue has a high concentration of uncoupling protein-1 (UCP-1) (thermogenin protein) in the inner mitochondrial membrane. UCP-1 is a transmembrane porin, which gives the protons an easy direct path into the matrix. This dissolves the electrochemical gradient and prevents ATP synthesis. This proton flow is instead dissipated as heat, a mechanism also known as nonshivering thermogenesis. Brown fat is multilocular and has more mitochondria and thermogenin protein making it optimal for generating heat. Brown fat is highly concentrated in neonates and hibernating animals.

How could a single point mutation in the cystic fibrosis transmembrane regulator (CFTR), a membrane transporter protein that transports sugars, chloride, cations, and other peptides, result in the pathogenesis of cystic fibrosis?

The most common mutation in CF is the ΔF508 mutation, which is the loss of the amino acid phenylalanine. The ER quality control apparatus recognizes the protein as misfolded and prevents the protein from reaching the cell membrane. This leads to osmotic imbalances and thick, sticky mucus plugs that cannot be removed by cilia.

CHAPTER 20

Vesicle Transport

THE SECRETORY PATHWAY

How are proteins identified and admitted to the secretory pathway?

An **N-terminal signal sequence** is recognized by the signal recognition particle (SRP) and admitted to the secretory pathway. This critical step is mediated by the Sec 61 complex, a protein channel, responsible for protein translocation and insertion of integral membrane proteins into the lipid bilayer.

Why does the sequence of growth hormone in the human genome encode a 217 amino acid protein while the secreted form of growth hormone is only 191 amino acids?

Proteins destined to enter the secretory pathway are labeled with an N-terminal signal sequence of roughly 25 amino acids that ensures they are recognized by SRP and translocated across the rough endoplasmic reticulum (RER) membrane. During or immediately following translocation, this sequence is cleaved by signal peptidase, hence shortening the length of the final secreted product.

What is meant by the prefixes *pre* and *pro* in the expression pre-pro-insulin?

The prefix *pre* specifies that the protein contains a cleavable N-terminal signal sequence competent for translocation. *Pro* indicates that the peptide will be further cleaved by an additional protease before it is biologically active. Pro-proteins are often stored in this inactive state to increase their storage shelf life or to prevent deleterious enzymatic activity in the wrong cellular location.

Secretory proteins can belong to either the constitutive secretory pathway or the regulated secretory pathway. What are the general characteristics of these pathways, and how are the unique fates of these proteins distinguished in the trans Golgi?

The pathways for constitutive and regulated protein secretion are initially identical but diverge in the trans Golgi apparatus. See Table 20.1.

Table 20.1 Constitutive Pathway Versus Regulated Pathway

	Constitutive (Default) Secretory Pathway	Regulated Secretory Pathway
Proteins	Proteins required at relatively constant levels for housekeeping and homeostatic functions, eg, serum proteins (albumin from hepatocytes) and components of the extracellular matrix (collagen from fibroblasts)	Proteins that are dangerous in excess or ineffective if not properly coordinated; eg, protein hormones (ACTH from the pituitary gland) and degradative enzymes (chymotrypsin from pancreas)
Target delivery	Delivered to the surface via exocytosis (constitutive)	Stored in the cytoplasm as secretory vesicles (regulated)

Ehlers-Danlos syndrome (EDS) is a heterogeneous group of connective tissue disorders with a defect in collagen or its synthesis. It is characterized by hyperextensible skin, easy bruising, and loose joints. List some proteins and enzymes that are commonly mutated in EDS.

Lysyl hydroxylase: hydroxylated lysine residues are important in cross-linking collagen, which provides tensile strength. This is EDS type VI, characterized by neonatal kyphoscoliosis with muscle hypotonia at birth.

Procollagen peptidase: upon secretion, triple helical procollagen is cleaved by peptidase, which initiates fibril assembly.

Collagen mutations: EDS type IV is a deficiency of type III collagen, classically associated with susceptibility to aneurysm formations, aortic dissections, and visceral perforation.

VESICLE FORMATION AND TRANSPORT

What division of labor exists between coatomer-coated (COP) and clathrin-coated vesicles?

Clathrin-coated vesicles are part of the regulated secretory pathway. Coatomer-coated vesicles transport proteins through the constituitive pathway. See Table 20.2.

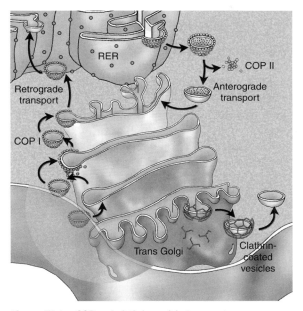

Figure 20.1   COP and clathrin vesicle transport.

Table 20.2 COP Versus Clathrin-Coated Vesicles

Vesicle Coat	Coatomer-Coated (COP) Vesicles	Clathrin Coated Vesicles
Pathways	Constitutive secretory pathways: COP I: retrograde transport (Golgi to ER) COP II: anterograde transport (ER to Golgi, etc); unregulated transport operations (eg, bulk flow of ECM constituents to the cell surface).	Receptor-mediated endocytosis and regulated transport of vesicles leaving the trans Golgi network (TGN) for other intracellular organelles.

Considerable structural homology exists between the components surrounding both COP and clathrin-coated vesicles. What do these vesicle coatings contribute that is so essential for efficient transport?

Vesicular fusion is most efficient for highly curved membranes, which are thermodynamically stabilized by these coats. Coat proteins also help to concentrate cargo, recruit appropriate and exclude inappropriate cargo, and accelerate budding.

Much like the delivery of mail using zip codes, proteins in the secretory pathway are labeled with molecular signals to ensure safe arrival. What are the appropriate signals for localization to the:

Endoplasmic reticulum (ER) targeting/ER retention

KDEL

Golgi targeting/Golgi retention

A single transmembrane α helix, three amino acids shorter than most helices of integral plasma membrane proteins

Lysosomal targeting

Mannose-6-phosphate

Apical membrane of polarized cells

Glycosylphosphatidylinositol (GPI) anchor, N- (added in the ER) and O-glycans (added in the Golgi)

Basolateral membrane of polarized cells

NPXY, LL

Clostridial neurotoxins (tetanus, botulinum) are metalloproteases that destroy synaptic vesicle fusion machinery and thus prevent neurotransmitter release. What are the three essential components of the SNARE complex, and how do they enable fusion?

SNAP-25, syntaxin, and synaptobrevin (also called VAMP for vesicle-associated membrane protein) are essential for vesicle fusion. Synaptobrevin resides in the vesicle membrane, whereas SNAP-25 and syntaxin reside on the target plasma membrane. When intracellular calcium rises, the α helical coiled coils of this complex zip together to join the adjacent membranes.

In the interest of energetic economy and signaling efficiency, some receptors taken up by ligand during receptor-mediated endocytosis are promptly returned to the cell surface. How is this receptor recycling accomplished?

Early endosomes filled with ligand-bound receptors are acidified by vacuolar H^+-ATPase. This acidic environment stimulates ligand-receptor dissociation to form the compartment for uncoupling of receptor and ligand (CURL), a structure in which receptors cluster in membrane outpouchings that pinches off and recycles reusable receptors to the cell surface.

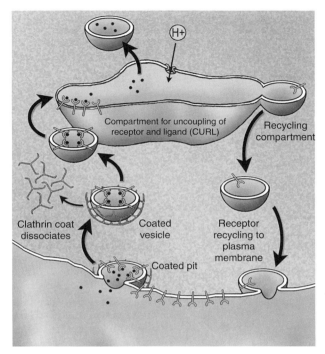

Figure 20.2   Receptor recycling.

TYPES OF ENDOCYTOSIS

What are the four main mechanisms cells used to take up material?

1. Transcytosis
2. Pinocytosis
3. Phagocytosis
4. Receptor-mediated endocytosis

External epithelial surfaces of the body, such as the respiratory and digestive tracts, are susceptible to infection and therefore protected by the humoral immune system. How is it possible for plasma cells in the lamina propria to contribute immunoglobulins to the apical (luminal) surface of epithelia?

Transcytosis. Plasma cells secrete IgA dimers complexed with a **J-chain,** a structure recognized by poly-Ig receptors on the basolateral surface of the epithelium. Once bound, the receptor-immunoglobulin complex is taken up in a clathrin-coated pit via endocytosis and transported to the apical surface of the epithelium. Fusion is accompanied by proteolysis of the poly-Ig receptor, which releases a peptide fragment appropriately named secretory component.

How is phagocytosis different from receptor-mediated endocytosis?

Phagocytosis is actin-dependent, sporadic, and occurs in specialized cells, for example, immune cells. **Receptor-mediated endocytosis** is clathrin coat–dependent, is involved in the uptake of specific material, and the cell can be refractory to the ligand if the specific receptor is degraded.

Describe phagocytosis of bacteria by macrophages.

Phagocytes have surface receptors that identify microbes coated with antibodies (eg, IgG) and complement proteins (eg, C3b). C3b is also known as an opsonin, and the process of coating the bacterium to render it susceptible to phagocytosis is called opsonization. Following uptake, the engulfed particle is called a phagosome until fusion with lysosomes, transforming it into a phagolysosome.

Give examples of exocytosis.

1. Pancreatic acinar cells secrete digestive enzymes (eg, lipase, amylase) in response to cholecystokinin.
2. Intestinal cells synthesize fat droplets from fatty acids and monoglycerides and exocytose the fat into lymph vessels, called lacteals.
3. At synaptic sites, two neurons will release neurotransmitters through exocytosis.

In receptor-mediated endocytosis, the ligand-receptor complex has a choice of four fates. Give examples of each of the following scenarios:

Recycled receptors and degraded ligands

Low-density lipoprotein (LDL) receptor and LDL

Recycled receptors and ligands

Transferrin receptor and transferrin, which delivers iron

Degraded receptors and ligands

Epidermal growth factor (EGF) and its tyrosine kinase EGF receptor; significance of receptor degradation is to abate the cell's capacity to respond to the ligand and to downregulate the intracellular signal cascade

Transported receptors and ligands (eg, transcytosis)

Secretory IgA and poly-Ig receptor

CLINICAL CORRELATES AND VIGNETTES

A 19 yo athlete presents to a dermotologist with xanthomas on her knees and feet. Bloodwork reveals an elevated cholesterol level. She also c/o blurred vision. What are the diagnosis and the molecular etiology of her condition?

Familial hypercholesterolemia is a defect of the LDL receptor. Defects include abnormal receptor synthesis, impaired recognition or affinity of apolipoprotein B-100 on the LDL surface, disrupted internalization via receptor-mediated endocytosis, or deficient recycling of receptor following internalization. Failure to take up LDL particles leads to high cholesterol, accelerated atherosclerosis, coronary heart disease, and buildup of cholesterol in the cornea and just below the skin.

A patient with no history of dyslipidemias is diagnosed with hypothyroidism and 3 months later with hypercholesterolemia. What is the link between these conditions?

The presence of T_3 enhances the interaction of apolipoprotein B-100 with LDL-R leading to degradation of cholesterol. Chronically low levels of thyroid hormone thus often lead to accumulation of cholesterol in the blood.

A patient with manic depression is treated with lithium and soon develops lethargy, constipation, and flaking skin. At 3 μg/dL, his T4 levels are remarkably low. What is the problem?

Lithium carbonate inhibits vesicle fusion in the thyroid, thereby causing hypothyroidism. It inhibits fusion of vesicles containing free thyroid hormones T_3 and T_4 at the basolateral surface. Because the drug is so effective for manic depression, therapy is usually continued and exogenous thyroid hormone is administered.

A 10 yo unvaccinated boy is playing in his garage when he steps on a rusty old nail. Over the next 3 days, he begins to feel tingling in the painful area around the puncture site. One week later, he presents to the local emergency department with a headache, a stiff jaw, and spastic paralysis of his left leg. What was the mechanism of the toxin producing his symptoms?

Tetanus is a condition caused by *Clostridium tetani*. The tetanus toxin is a metalloprotease that cleaves synaptobrevin, a protein that is critical for neurotransmitter release. Acting on the inhibitory interneurons of Renshaw in the spinal cord, tetanus toxin prevents the release of glycine onto the lower motor neurons of the ventral horn. Consequently, any stimulus leads to uncontrollable muscle spasms and exaggerated reflexes.

A 47 yo F suddenly begins to have difficulty swallowing food during dinner. She is brought to the hospital and a few hours later, she develops dysarthria and diplopia. On examination, she is alert, oriented, and able to follow commands. Her forced vital capacity is 500 mL, and she is intubated. She is afebrile, tachycardic, and normotensive. Facial sensation is intact, but bifacial paresis is present. Motor strength in proximal upper and lower extremities is 4 out of 5. What is the mechanism of this disease?

Botulism. The botulinum toxin from *Clostridium botulinum* blocks ACh release in the autonomic and peripheral NMJs. It causes an acute onset of flaccid paralysis, b/l neuropathies, such as bulbar paresis and a symmetric descending weakness, and life-threatening respiratory arrest. The patient often presents with a clear sensorium, is afebrile, and has no sensory deficits except blurry vision. Other classic presentations include a "floppy baby" after ingesting honey with spores in it or after eating improperly canned foods.

You are shocked to observe a patient consume more than a liter of water. She admits to drinking about 15 L of water each day and waking repeatedly in the night to drink and urinate. She is refractory to desmopressin acetate (dDAVP) (vasopressin) therapy. What is her diagnosis?

Nephrogenic diabetes insipidus (DI) is a condition where the kidneys fail to respond to antidiuretic hormone (ADH). ADH normally acts on the V2 receptors in the thick ascending limb of the nephron to traffic vesicle-stored aquaporin 2 (AQP2) water channels to the cell surface; this allows for water reabsorption and secretion of concentrated urine.

CHAPTER 21

Cell Cycle Division

CELL CYCLE

What are the five stages of the cell cycle? What occurs at each stage?   See Table 21.1

Table 21.1 Cell Cycle Phases

Phase	Purpose of Phase
G_1 (Gap 1)	Cell growth; RNA and protein synthesis
G_0	Resting
S (Synthesis)	DNA synthesis and replication
G_2 (Gap 2)	Surveillance of replicated DNA to ensure it has doubled; specialized protein synthesis required for mitosis to proceed
M phase	Mitosis and cytokinesis
Interphase	Chromosome replication

Describe the different checkpoints in the cell cycle.   See Table 21.2

Table 21.2 Cell Cycle Checkpoints

Checkpoint	
G_1 checkpoint	p53 causes G_1 arrest when damaged DNA is detected. If the DNA damage cannot be corrected, apoptosis ensues.
S-phase checkpoint	Checks for DNA damage and ensures fidelity of the replicated DNA. The cell monitors for presence of Okazaki fragments on the lagging strand during DNA replication.
G_2 checkpoint	Damaged DNA will arrest cells in the G_2 phase.
M checkpoint (spindle-attachment checkpoint)	Ensures that the spindle fibers are attached to the kinetochores.

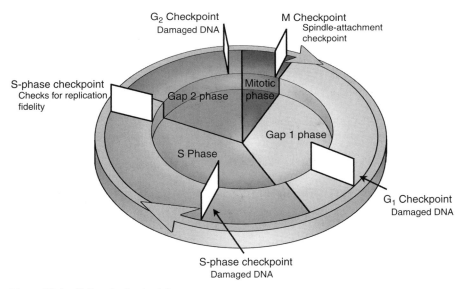

Figure 21.1   Cell cycle checkpoints.

What stage of the cell cycle would a random epithelial cell most likely be in? Bone marrow cell? Nerve cell? Muscle cell? Lymphocyte?

1. Epithelial cells and bone marrow cells: G_1 phase; they constantly replicate to replenish dying cells and would likely be in the longest phase of the cell cycle.
2. Nerve and muscle cells: G_0 phase; they are nondividing and reside in a quiescent state.
3. Lymphocytes: G_0 phase unless they are antigenically stimulated to reenter the cell cycle.

Name three gene products involved in the checkpoints.

1. **p53**: senses DNA damage and can induce apoptosis
2. **Ataxia telangiectasia mutated (ATM)**: detects DNA damage, especially double-strand breaks
3. **Mitotic arrest deficient (MAD)**: involved in the spindle checkpoint

Discuss how the spindle checkpoint works.

Each chromosome is associated with a kinetochore, a protein that links the chromosome to microtubule polymers from the mitotic spindle. *MAD* genes encode kinetochore proteins that ensure chromosomal attachment to a spindle fiber. MAD remains on unattached kinetochores and blocks entry into anaphase.

Infection with the human T-cell leukemia virus-1 (HTLV-1) leads to adult T-cell leukemia (ATL) in about 5% of its victims. HTLV-1 encodes a protein, called Tax, which binds and inhibits the MAD protein. How would this manifest in cancer cells?

Leukemic cells in these patients show many chromosome abnormalities, including aneuploidy, due to abnormal alignments and attachments of spindle fibers.

Each cell cycle phase has an associated cyclin and cyclin-dependent kinase (cdk) complex. Cyclin levels oscillate with each phase, but cdk levels are stable throughout. Describe each cyclin-cdk complex for each cell cycle phase.

See Table 21.3

Table 21.3 Cyclin-Dependent Kinases and Cyclins

Cyclin	Kinase	Function
D	Cdk4, Cdk6	G_1-Cdk: progression past restriction point at G1/S boundary
E, A	Cdk2	G_1/S-Cdk, S-Cdk: initiation of DNA synthesis in the S phase
B	Cdk1	M-Cdk: transition from G_2 to M

How are cdks regulated?

Cdks are controlled by inhibitors. Cdk activation occurs only after complexing with the appropriate cyclin. When activated, cdk phosphorylates proteins that control progression in the cell cycle.

MITOSIS

What is the difference between mitosis and cytokinesis?

Mitosis is nuclear division (microtubule-based), and cytokinesis is cytoplasmic division (actin-based).

What are the stages of mitosis and the defining features of each?

1. **Prophase**: chromatin condenses into chromosomes, nucleolus disappears, and mitotic spindle forms.
2. **Prometaphase**: nuclear envelope disintegrates, and spindle fibers attach to the kinetochores of the chromosomes.
3. **Metaphase**: homologous chromosomes line up midway between the poles of the spindle (metaphase plate) and can be karyotyped.
4. **Anaphase**: sister chromatids separate.
5. **Telophase**: nuclear envelope reforms around the chromosomes, chromosomes decondense, and cytokinesis begins.

A cell grown in culture is treated with colchicine, a reagent that blocks the formation of spindle microtubules. In which phase will the cells be arrested?

Prophase. The cell will be unable to proceed to metaphase without spindle formation, which is carried out by microtubule polymerization.

Name cancer drugs that are specific to the phases of mitosis.

See Table 21.4

Table 21.4 Cancer Drugs

Phase of Mitosis	Drug
S	6-mercaptopurine, 6-thioguanine, cytarabine, hydroxyurea, methotrexate, 5-FU
G_2	bleomycin, etoposide, doxorubicin
M	vinblastine, paclitaxel, vincristine
G_0	Alkylating agents (eg, cyclophosphamide, cisplatin, nitrosoureas, procarbazine), dacarbazine, busulfan

MEIOSIS

What is the function of meiosis?

To produce haploid gametes from one diploid germ cell. In spermatogenesis, four haploid spermatozoa are formed; in oogenesis, one haploid ovum is formed. The other haploid cells, called polar bodies, are resorbed. Meiosis is necessary for sexual reproduction.

What is the meaning of

Diploid

Diploid (2n): having two sets of chromosomes, for example, most human cells

Haploid

Haploid (1n): having one set of chromosomes, for example, human gametes

Aneuploid

Aneuploid: having an abnormal number of chromosomes, for example, in trisomy 21, three copies of chromosome 21 are present instead of two

How many chromosomes are present in the cells at the end of meiosis I and meiosis II?

Meiosis I is a reductional division, and meiosis II is an equatorial division. At the end of meiosis I, homologous chromosomes separate to create two haploid cells (reduced from its diploid state), for example, 23 chromosomes in human cells. At the end of meiosis II, chromatids separate, maintaining the haploid number of chromosomes.

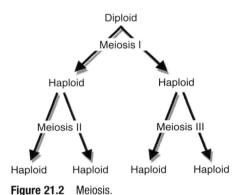

Figure 21.2 Meiosis.

How does meiosis result in genetic variation and increase its genetic diversity?

Crossing-over during meiosis I enables gene exchange between segments of homologous chromosomes.

Independent assortment during meiosis I results in random distribution of maternal and paternal chromosomes to the gametes.

APOPTOSIS

How does apoptosis differ from cell necrosis?

Apoptosis is noninflammatory, programmed cell death. By contrast, **cell necrosis** results from acute injury leading to **inflammation**.

Contrast morphologic characteristics of apoptosis with cell necrosis.

See Table 21.5

Table 21.5 Apoptosis and Cell Necrosis

	Apoptosis	Cell Necrosis
Morphologic characteristics	1. Cell shrinkage 2. Nuclear fragmentation 3. Chromatin condensation (pyknosis) 4. Discontinuation of nuclear membrane (karyorrhexis) 5. Cellular fragmentation into membrane-enclosed apoptotic bodies 6. Cell membrane blebbing 7. Phagocytosis of remnants	1. Cell swelling 2. Enzymatic digestion 2. Protein denaturation 3. Cell lysis 4. Release of intracellular components 5. Inflammatory process

Describe some extracellular signals that induce apoptosis.

Absence of growth factors, absence of proper extracellular matrix (ECM) contacts, viral infections, and presence of Fas ligand (FasL)

What are the main functions of apoptosis? Give examples.

Development
1. Embryogenesis: fetal development of fingers and toes requires apoptosis of intervening tissues between digits.

Maintenance of adult tissues and destruction of infected or damaged cells.
1. Cytotoxic T-lymphocytes kill virally infected cells by inducing apoptosis.
2. Cells with irreversible DNA damage commit suicide; p53 is an inducer of apoptosis.
3. Menstruation.

Name the triggers for the two different pathways of apoptosis—the mitochondrial pathway and the cell death receptor pathway.

Cell death receptor pathway (extrinsic pathway): FasL and its surface receptor (also known as CD95), TNF-α (tumor necrosis factor-α), and TNF-β (lymphotoxin) and its receptor

Mitochondrial pathway (intrinsic pathway): DNA damage (from UV light, x-rays, chemotherapeutic drugs), accumulation of oxidants within cells, accumulation of improperly folded proteins

Describe the key molecules involved in the intrinsic pathway.

Intracellular damage leads the **Bcl-2** protein on the outer mitochondrial membrane to activate protein **Bax**. Bax functions to damage the outer mitochondrial membrane. This causes **cytochrome c**, an electron carrier protein, to leak into the cytosol. Cytochrome c binds **Apaf-1**, an adaptor protein. This complex is known as an **apoptosome**, which binds and activates **caspase-9**, leading to the caspase cascade.

Describe the key molecules involved in this extrinsic apoptotic pathway.

The binding of **FasL** to its receptor results in trimerization. This complex recruits adaptor proteins, which aids in aggregating **caspase-8**. This leads to the caspase cascade.

CANCER

What is an oncogene?

It is a mutated form of a protooncogene, a gene typically involved in **cell growth** or **proliferation**. The type of mutation is usually a **gain-of-function** (activating) mutation of a **single gene copy**, which has dominant effects and results in constitutive cell proliferation.

Name examples of oncogenes and their associated tumors.

See Table 21.6

Table 21.6 Oncogenes and Tumors

Oncogene	Associated Tumor
c-myc	Burkitt's lymphoma
bcl-2	Follicular and undifferentiated lymphomas, chronic myelogenous lymphoma
erb-B2	Breast, ovarian, and gastric carcinomas
ras	Colon cancer
fos	Osteogenic sarcoma
l-myc	Lung tumor
ret	Multiple endocrine neoplasia type II
MEN1	Multiple endocrine neoplasia type I

Describe types of mutations that convert a protooncogene to an oncogene.

Typically, mutations result in an overproduction of normal protein or a hyperactive protein.

Point mutation or partial deletion: creates a constitutively active protein.

Chromosomal translocation: protooncogene has a constitutively active promoter.

Genomic amplification: normal protein is overabundantly expressed.

The development of cancer from benign to malignant stages may be a result of sequential mutations. Colorectal cancer is a classic example. Often one key mutation triggers an initial tumor cell population and, with an increased rate of proliferation, successive mutations create a variant cell population that rapidly takes over. Describe some key characteristics of cancer cells that may result from successive mutations.

The development of cancer requires the accumulation of multiple mutations.

Key characteristics of cancer cells include:
1. Defects in apoptotic signals and cell regulatory signals
2. Genetically unstable
3. No proliferative restriction
4. Ability to dedifferentiate
5. Invasive
6. Ability to metastasize
7. Angiogenesis
8. Ability to hide from the immune system

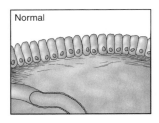
Normal

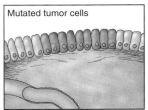
Mutated tumor cells

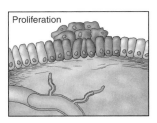
Proliferation

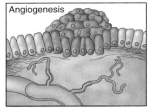
Angiogenesis

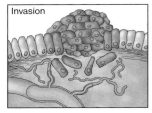
Invasion

Figure 21.3   Cancer progression and characteristics.

What types of molecules are protooncogenes?

Growth factors: for example, *sis* gene; encodes platelet-derived growth factor.

Growth factor receptors: for example, *erbB* gene; encodes epidermal growth factor receptors.

Protein kinases: for example, *abl* gene; translocation to *bcr* on chromosome 22 results in chronic myelogenous leukemia.

Nuclear proteins/transcription factors: for example, *fos* gene; mutation results in osteogenic sarcoma.

What is a tumor suppressor gene?

Also known as antioncogenes, these genes typically regulate mitosis. They require **loss-of-function** (inactivating) **mutations in both copies of the gene**, and act recessively, leading to **unregulated cell growth**.

Describe some genetic mutations, resulting in tumor suppressor gene inactivation.

1. Nondisjunction leading to chromosome loss
2. Deletion
3. Point mutation
4. Epigenetic changes leading to methylation of the promoter, resulting in gene silencing

Name examples of tumor suppressor genes and their associated tumors.

See Table 21.7.

Table 21.7 Tumor Suppressor Genes and Tumors

Tumor Suppressor Gene	Chromosome	Associated Tumor
rb	13q	Retinoblastoma, osteosarcoma
BRCA1 and 2	17q, 13q	Breast and ovarian cancer
p53	17p	Many cancers, including Li-Fraumeni syndrome
p16	9p	Melanoma
APC	5q	Colorectal cancer
WT1	11q	Wilm's tumor
NF1	17q	Neurofibromatosis type 1
NF2	22q	Neurofibromatosis type 2
DPC	18q	Pancreatic cancer
DCC	18q	Colon cancer

You have discovered a new protein called Bob. You have shown that knocking out both copies of the *bob* gene eventually leads to rapid proliferation of cells. Describe roles that Bob may play in cells.

The *bob* gene is a tumor suppressor gene. Potential roles for the Bob protein include:

1. **Transcriptional repressors**: Bob could inhibit the transcription of genes needed in the S-phase (eg, *wt1* gene; Wilm's tumor).
2. **Checkpoint protein**: Bob could monitor the integrity of DNA and arrest the cell cycle in the event of DNA damage (eg, *p53* gene; Li-Fraumeni syndrome, *atm* gene).
3. **Cdk inhibitor**: Bob could inhibit the cell cycle kinases, the loss of which would release the brake on the cell cycle (eg, *cdk-p16* gene).
4. **GTPase proteins**: Bob could remove the GTP from activated Ras, thereby inactivating the cell cycle stimulator (eg, *NF-1* gene; von Recklinghausen disease).
5. **Ubiquitin protein ligase**: Bob could add a degradation tag, ubiquitin, to proteins that stimulate growth factor production (eg, *vhl* or *von Hippel-Lindau* gene; hemangiomas).

What does the protein p53 do?

It **senses DNA damage** and stops progression of the cell cycle in G_1, allowing for repair. It plays a role in apoptosis of irreparably damaged cells. p53 protects cells from mutations that may lead to uncontrolled proliferation; it is a tumor suppressor.

How does p53 halt the cell cycle?

p53 induces **p21** binding and inactivation of the **cyclin E/cdk2 complex**, thereby halting cell cycle progression.

Tumors with mutated *p53* genes generally respond poorly to chemotherapy, while tumors with intact *p53* have good results with chemotherapy. Explain.

Chemotherapy induces DNA damage. In cells with intact p53, the *p53* gene product halts the cell cycle until the DNA damage is repaired or initiates cell apoptosis. A cell with mutated *p53* continues to survive and proliferate despite DNA damage.

One strategy for anticancer chemotherapy is to target cells in mitosis. Describe three potential targets to block cells in mitosis. What would be the likely effect on the cell?

Possible targets include regulatory proteins that cause a cell to exit mitosis or components of the mitotic checkpoint pathway. See Table 21.8

Table 21.8 Drug Targets

Drug	Target	Effect on Cell
Taxol	Microtubules	Inhibits depolymerization of microtubules. Mitotic checkpoint activated → Apoptosis.
Colchicine	Tubulin	Blocks polymerization of microtubules → Unable to form mitotic spindle → Mitotic checkpoint activated → Apoptosis.
Vinblastine or vincristine	Tubulin and microtubules	Blocks microtubule depolymerization at low concentrations and polymerization at high concentrations → Blocks dividing cells in mitosis → Apoptosis.

Why are chemotherapeutic drugs inevitably toxic above a certain dose? Which cells would be affected in toxicity?

Toxicity is inevitable since the process of mitosis is the same in cancer cells and in dividing cells. The cells most likely to be affected are the rapidly dividing cells in the bone marrow and GI tract.

Chemotherapeutic agents induce apoptosis relatively simultaneously in a large population of cells. This has the potential to result in tumor lysis syndrome (TLS), particularly in the case of lymphomas. What laboratory abnormalities can be detected in TLS?

Hyperkalemia

Hyperphosphatemia

Hyperuricemia

Hyperuricosuria

Hypocalcemia

CLINICAL CORRELATES AND VIGNETTES

What abnormality in the meiotic process is responsible for Down syndrome?

Down's syndrome, or **trisomy 21**, is the result of **meiosis I nondisjunction**, or the failure of homologous chromosomes to separate during meiotic division, resulting in an extra chromosome.

Why does "debulking" a tumor improve the efficacy of chemotherapeutics?

"Debulking" involves removing a significant mass from a solid tumor. When a tumor is debulked, many of the remaining tumor cells transition from G_0 to G_1 due to a relative increase in the availability of nutrition, oxygen, and growth factors. This process is important because chemotherapeutics and radiation therapy primarily target actively dividing cells. A larger proportion of the tumor will now respond to chemotherapeutics or radiation therapy.

How does human papillomavirus (HPV) interact with p53 to cause cervical cancer?

HPV **degrades p53**, which normally halts the cell cycle by inactivating the cyclin E/cdk 2 complex. This can lead to uncontrolled cellular proliferation, which is the case in cervical cancer.

What does the *rb* (retinoblastoma) gene do?

The *rb* gene is a **tumor suppressor gene** whose protein product binds and **inactivates E2F**, a transcription factor that activates cell proliferation genes.

The protooncogene *erbB-2* encodes a receptor protein tyrosine kinase, HER2. Oncogenic HER2 is amplified and expressed at high levels in about 30% of breast cancers. Elevated expression of HER2 is characteristic of rapidly progressing metastatic cancers with a poor prognosis. How would you design a new treatment based on this information?

ErbB-2 protein has served as the first oncogene target for a new FDA-approved anticancer drug. The drug, Herceptin is approved for clinical use in patients with HER2 positive breast cancer. It is an antibody designed to bind and inactivate the oncogenic HER2 receptor protein tyrosine kinase. It thus selectively targets and kills tumor cells that overexpress HER2.

A 26 yo M athlete c/o itchiness between his toes. On exam, the skin on his feet is scaly with erythematous, papulovesicular lesions. He is concerned it will spread to his groin. What is his diagnosis and what is the mechanism of the oral antifungal that is prescribed?

Tinea pedis is a fungal infection, and **griseofulvin** inhibits microtubule function, thereby disrupting fungal cell mitosis in metaphase.

A 30 yo alcoholic M c/o epigastric abdominal pain radiating to his back. He reports fever, anorexia, and N/V for 48 hours. On exam, his abdomen is tender, rigid, and has diminished bowel sounds. What are you concerned about, and what type of cellular injury leads to the inflammatory response?

In **acute pancreatitis,** pancreatic enzymes, such as lipase, are activated and released into the tissue. This is called **fat necrosis,** leading to an inflammatory response rich in neutrophils.

A 4-week-old infant comes to your office. The parents report that the infant's eyes do not seem to be moving in the same direction. You perform a fundoscopic eye examination and find white reflections in both eyes. What is the most likely diagnosis, and what is the probable etiology behind this patient's condition?

The white reflection on examination of the pupils, called leukocoria, makes **retinoblastoma**, familial type, the most likely diagnosis. Retinoblastoma occurs in two forms. In the sporadic type, both genes undergo sporadic mutations and develop into a unilateral tumor. This illustrates the "two hit hypothesis" where two random chance mutations occur and often affects one eye in early childhood.

In the familial type, multiple tumors occur in both eyes during infancy. All of the cells are heterozygote for the mutated copy of the *rb* gene. These cells are predisposed to becoming cancerous when a somatic mutation occurs in the other copy; loss of the normal gene, called "loss of heterozygosity," leads to tumor formation.

A 67 yo F c/o a 15 lb weight loss over 3 months and anorexia. Upon further questioning, she reports pruritus, acholic stools, and dark urine. Her physical exam is significant for icteric sclerae, jaundice, and epigastric tenderness. An abdominal CT scan reveals a mass in the pancreatic head. See Figure 21.4. What is a common tumor suppressor gene that leads to this pathology?

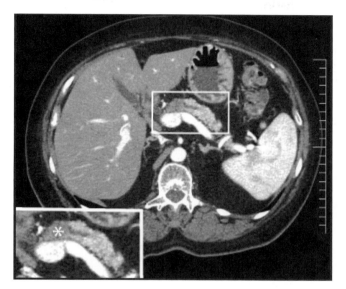

Figure 21.4   Pancreatic head mass.

The *DPC* **gene** (18q chromosome), a **tumor suppressor gene**, is commonly mutated in **pancreatic adenocarcinoma**. She has signs of painless, obstructive, jaundice. Her CT scan reveals a pancreatic head mass.

CHAPTER 22

Extracellular Matrix and Cell-to-Cell Interactions

INTRODUCTION

Define connective tissue.

Organization of different cells together

What is an organ?

Organ = connective tissue + extracellular matrix (ECM)

Why is the ECM important?

1. Acts as a physical scaffold
2. Matrix for cellular migration
3. Mediates cell-to-cell signaling

Name the components of a proteoglycan.

Glycosaminoglycans (GAGs) covalently linked to a core protein

What is the ECM composed of? How is the ECM produced?

The ECM is composed of a variety of proteoglycans and fibrous proteins (eg, collagen, elastin, fibronectin, laminin), which are produced and secreted into the extracellular space by local cells, such as fibroblasts.

What is another name for the ECM of epithelial cells?

Basal lamina

Degradation of the ECM is important for many cellular processes. Give an example where the ECM is degraded.

Cellular migration. Leukocytes migrate through the basal lamina of a blood vessel to access the site of an infection.

How is ECM degradation regulated?

Proteolytic enzymes, eg, serine proteases and matrix metalloproteases.

Three mechanisms of regulation include:
1. **Local activity**: most proteases, found in inactive forms, are activated when needed (eg, plasminogen and plasmin).
2. Confined by **cell surface receptors**: cell surface receptors bind proteases thereby localizing degradation.
3. **Secrete inhibitors**: protease inhibitors prevent proteases from degrading beyond the designated area (eg, serine protease inhibitors known as serpins).

GLYCOPROTEINS

Glycosaminoglycan (GAG) chains occupy large amounts of space and form hydrated gels that can support high pressures. They are an integral component of joints. How does their structure enable them to resist compressive forces?

GAG chains are **strongly negatively charged**, attracting osmotically active cations, especially Na^+. This causes water to be pulled into the matrix creating a swelling pressure that allows the matrix to resist compressive forces. In the knee joint, the cartilage matrix made with GAGs can support hundreds of atmospheres of pressure.

Hyaluronan is considered the simplest of the GAG molecules. What is the role of hyaluronan in embryogenesis?

Hyaluronan is an important space filler in embryogenesis. Like other GAGs, a small amount can expand with water and occupy a large volume. Hyaluronan creates a cell-free space for cells, which can migrate during organ development. Once the migration is complete, excess hyaluronan is degraded by hyaluronidase.

Why are proteoglycans an important component of the ECM?

1. Form a **porous matrix** to regulate cell movement
2. Act as **transmembrane coreceptors** for growth factors
3. **Bind and regulate activities of other secreted proteins** (eg, immobilize protein and restrict range of action or protect protein from degradation)
4. Act as a **link between the ECM and cytoskeleton**

What is the function of the proteoglycan syndecan-1?

Transmembrane protein that **binds chemokines**. It is released when epithelia are damaged. The diffusing gradient of syndecan-1 acts as a chemotactic gradient that attracts neutrophils to the inflamed site.

FIBERS

Collagens are the major proteins of the extracellular matrix. What are the main types of collagen found in connective tissues?

See Table 22.1

Table 22.1 Types of Collagen

Collagen	Tissue Distribution	Synthesizing Cell	Main Function
Collagen I	Bone, dermis, tendon, sclera, fibrous ligaments, fascias, late wound repair	Fibroblast, osteoblast, odontoblast, chondroblast	Resistance against tension
Collagen II	Hyaline cartilage, elastic cartilage, vertebral disc	Chondroblast	Resistance to periodic pressure
Collagen III	Smooth muscle, skin, arteries, liver, spleen, kidneys, lungs, granulation tissue	Reticular cells, smooth muscle cells, Schwann cells, fibroblast, hepatocyte	Maintains structure in organs that can expand
Collagen IV	Epithelial and endothelial basal laminae and basement membrane	Endothelial and epithelial cells, muscle cells, Schwann cells	Support and filtration

Why is type IV collagen best suited to form part of the basal lamina?

Flexibility. Type IV collagens are not cleaved after secretion, and these uncleaved domains interact extracellularly and assemble into a more flexible, sheetlike network, an ideal shape for the thin mat that is the basal lamina.

In what types of tissues are elastic fibers most common?

Blood vessels, lungs, skin

Fibronectin is a ubiquitous glycoprotein in the ECM that circulates in the ECM and blood (soluble form) but is also found on cell surfaces (fibrillar form). What is its function?

Soluble form: substrate for blood coagulation factor VIII and functions in blood clotting and wound healing.

Fibrillar form: mediates migration by facilitating cell adhesion to the ECM by binding to integrin receptors. Transformed cells have reduced fibronectin, likely leading to decreased adherence to the ECM and increased mobility.

Basal laminae perform many diverse functions. Describe the role of the basal lamina in the kidney and in tissue regeneration.

The kidney glomerulus has a thick basal lamina that acts as a **filter** and prevents macromolecules from entering the urine.

In damaged tissues, the basal lamina provides a **scaffold for regeneration** to occur. Cells migrate to the basal lamina and begin the regeneration process.

CELLULAR JUNCTIONS AND CELL-CELL ADHESION

What are the three classes of cell junctions and their functions?

1. **Occluding junctions** (tight junctions) function as a seal preventing the passage of molecules between adjacent cells and help maintain cell polarity.
2. **Anchoring junctions** (focal adhesions, adherens junctions, desmosomes, hemidesmosomes) attach cells to neighboring cells or to the ECM.
3. **Communicating junctions** (gap junctions) regulate the passage of electrical or chemical signals directly from one cell to another.

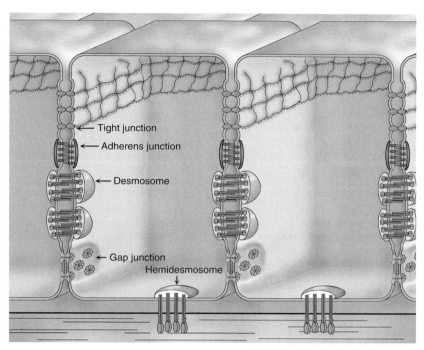

Figure 22.1   Cell junctions.

Epithelial cells can transiently alter tight junctions to allow greater flow of solutes and water. Why is this characteristic useful for a small intestinal cell?

Following meals, epithelia in the small intestine create breaches within their junctional barriers, allowing paracellular transport of solutes and water (eg, amino acids and monosaccharides) down their concentration gradient.

Where are anchoring junctions most abundant?

Parts of the body subjected to severe mechanical stress, such as the heart, muscle, and epidermis

How do adherens junctions aid in the formation of the neural tube?

They hold cells together and form a continuous adhesion belt encircling neighboring cells. In epithelial cells, a contractile bundle of actin filaments lies parallel to the adherens belt and attaches to the plasma membrane via intracellular anchor proteins. During neural tube formation, the contraction of actin filaments running with the adherens belt helps the epithelial sheet roll into a tube.

244 Deja Review: Histology & Cell Biology

What is the role of desmosomes in maintaining the integrity of the epidermis?

Anchoring junctions that hold skin keratinocytes together. Antibodies against desmosomal proteins can result in severe weakening of the epidermis, leading to a blistering skin disease called **pemphigus vulgaris**.

There are two forms of anchoring junctions made of proteins from either the cadherin or integrin families. How do these two types of junctions differ?

1. **Adherens junctions** and **desmosomes** are composed of transmembrane proteins from the **cadherin family**. They connect the plasma membrane from one cell to the plasma membrane of an adjacent cell.
2. **Focal adhesions** and **hemidesmosomes** are from the **integrin family**. They attach cells to the extracellular matrix. Bullous pemphigoid is an autoimmune disease against the hemidesmosome proteins.

Describe the function of gap junctions in cardiac myocytes and hepatocytes.

1. Cardiac myocytes are electrically coupled via gap junctions. Action potentials can spread rapidly without the delay that occurs at chemical synapses. This electrical coupling allows for synchronous heart contraction.
2. While some hepatocytes are innervated by sympathetic nerves, many hepatocytes are not. Gap junctions relay signals from the innervated hepatocytes to noninnervated hepatocytes, permitting messages to be transmitted to the whole liver.

What is the mechanism that allows the gap junction to switch between open and closed states?

Gap junctions are made of proteins from the connexin family. Six connexin transmembrane subunits form one channel or connexon. **Phosphorylation of connexins** is involved in the gating of gap junction channels.

Describe three signals that regulate gap junctions to oscillate between open and closed states.

1. Decreasing cytosolic **pH** reversibly decreases the permeability of gap junctions.
2. **Ca^{2+} levels**. Extracellular cations like Na^+ and Ca^{2+} can leak into injured cells. By closing the gap junctions, adjacent healthy cells are prevented from an increase in intracellular Ca^{2+} from the injured cell.
3. **Extracellular signals**. For example, dopamine reduces gap junction permeability in the retina in response to increased light intensity. This allows the retina to change from rod to cone photoreceptors, which are better suited to bright light.

What are cell adhesion molecules (CAMs)? Name some CAMs and their functions.

CAMs are cell surface proteins allowing cells to adhere to each other.

1. **Cadherins** primarily mediate Ca^{2+}-dependent cell-to-cell adhesion. There are many types of cadherins: E-cadherin—**e**pithelial cells; N-cadherin—**n**eurons, heart, skeletal muscle, lens, and fibroblasts.
2. **Selectins** are involved in transient Ca^{2+}-dependent cell-to-cell adhesion in the blood stream during inflammation. L-selectin is found on leukocytes, P-selectin is found on platelets, and E-selectin is found on endothelial cells.
3. **Neuronal cellular adhesion molecule** (**N-CAM**), present in most nerve cells, mediates Ca^{2+}-independent cell-cell adhesion.
4. **Intracellular adhesion molecule** (**I-CAM**), present on endothelial cells, binds to integrin on WBCs and attaches WBCs to endothelial cells.

What is an integrin?

Integrins are transmembrane cell adhesion proteins that act as matrix adhesion receptors. They bind the ECM to the cell's cytoskeleton or bind a cell to another cell (eg, WBCs).

What is their role?

Allow for transient adherence by binding their ligand with low affinity, thus preventing cells from being bound too tightly to the ECM.

How do selectins and integrins work together during white blood cell migration following tissue injury?

Selectins regulate a weak, reversible adhesion between leukocytes and vascular endothelium, which enables the leukocyte to roll along the endothelium, propelled by blood flow. The cells continue to roll until they activate **integrins, which form a stronger bond with the endothelium and allow adhesion**. The leukocyte then migrates out of the vasculature into the tissue.

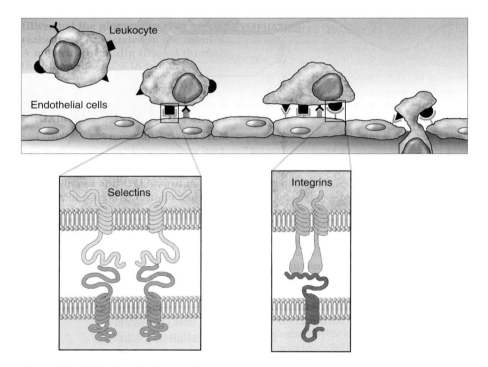

Figure 22.2   White blood cell margination.

CLINICAL CORRELATES AND VIGNETTES

How do cells in the small intestine maintain directional transport and prevent migration of transport proteins across the cell?

Tight junctions create a barrier to prevent the diffusion of transport proteins between the apical and basolateral surfaces of the plasma membrane. This maintains directional transport.

Design a cancer therapy that prevents tumor migration.

Tumor migration can be prevented with a **protease inhibitor**. Many cancers secrete proteases for tumor metastasis.

Many genetic diseases result from mutations that disrupt collagen formation. Describe some diseases.

1. **Osteogenesis imperfecta** is caused by mutations to **type I collagen** leading to easily fracturable, brittle bones. Hallmarks also include blue sclerae and hearing loss (middle ear bones are affected).
2. **Chondrodysplasias** are caused by mutations to **type II collagen**. They are characterized by abnormal cartilage causing bone and joint abnormalities.
3. **Ehlers-Danlos syndrome** (EDS) results from mutations to collagen or collagen synthesis; most common type of EDS is a deficiency of **type III collagen**. Tendency to bruise, hyperextensible skin, and moveable joints are the hallmarks of this disease. **Berry aneurysms** are associated.
4. **Alport syndrome** is caused by a mutation to **type IV collagen**. It is characterized by renal failure, deafness, and lens abnormalities.

Plasminogen is an example of a regulated extracellular proteolytic enzyme. How is it activated? Can it be activated by medications?

It is abundant in the blood in an inactive form and is **activated by tissue plasminogen activator (tPA), thrombin, fibrin, or factor XII** leading to **plasmin** formation and fibrinolysis. In the acute setting, **recombinant tPA** is given to patients who have had strokes or acute myocardial infarctions.

A 32 yo M presents to the ED with chest pain. On physical exam, the patient appears to have multiple bruises on his skin and hyperextensible joints. A CXR demonstrates a widened mediastinum. What is at the top of your differential diagnosis, and what is the histopathology behind the disease?

The patient has **Ehlers-Danlos syndrome IV**, which results in a deficiency in the production of **type III collagen.** It is an AD connective tissue disorder. For patients affected by this syndrome, spontaneous aortic rupture is the leading cause of death due to a propensity for aneurysms to form.

A neonate p/w six unique fractures within the first year of life. His parents cannot recall a serious accident in any of these incidents. Physical exam reveals blue sclerae, scoliosis, and poor hearing. What is the diagnosis and the molecular etiology of this condition?

Osteogenesis imperfecta (brittle bone disease). Many possible mutations exist, but most mutations are predominantly in the pro-α chains of **collagen type I**, which prevent the assembly of procollagen triple helices in the ER. Misfolded collagen aggregates in the ER initiate the unfolded protein response, which often leads to apoptosis of the stressed cell. Severely deleterious mutations completely prevent procollagen assembly and are embryonically lethal.

A 43 yo tall, slender M with long extremities p/w the worst headache of his life. A non-contrast head CT scan reveals a subarachnoid hemorrhage with a large aneurysm. For definitive treatment, he undergoes a cerebral angiogram, and the aneurysm is subsequently coiled. See Figure 22.3. What underlying genetic mutation predisposes the patient to aneurysms?

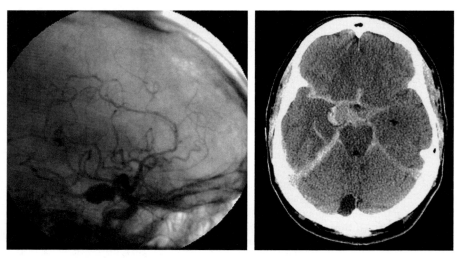

Figure 22.3   Coiled aneurysm.

His physical appearance suggests he has **Marfan's syndrome**, an AD disease with a mutation in the *fibrillin* gene. The fibrillin protein is essential for biogenesis and maintenance of elastin. Berry aneurysms are commonly associated with Marfan's syndrome, Autosomal Dominant Polycystic Kidney Disease (ADPKD), and Ehlers Danlos syndrome.

A 30 yo nonsmoking M presents to the ED with sudden sharp chest pain and shortness of breath. His PMHx and FHx are significant for chronic liver disease and emphysema. A CXR shows a large right-sided pneumothorax. See Figure 22.4. What is his underlying genetic disease, and what enzyme is altered?

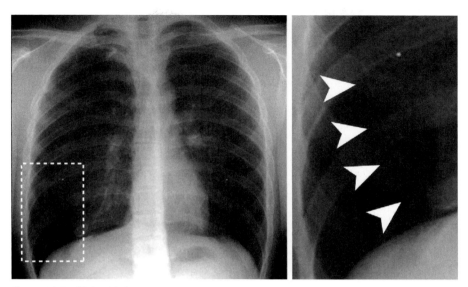

Figure 22.4   Right-sided pneumothorax.

α_1-**Antitrypsin deficiency** should be suspected in any young, nonsmoking individual (< 45 yo) with panacinar emphysema and liver disease. α_1-Antitrypsin is an inhibitor of the proteolytic enzyme **elastase**. Increased elastase activity leads to bullous changes, typically more prominent at the lung bases. Spontaneous rupture of the bullae can lead to pneumothoraces.

A 2 mo F infant p/w a 1-day h/o erythematous swelling and pain in the right cheek. Birth history included a late separation of the umbilical cord and treatment for an umbilical cord infection. Physical exam reveals a small febrile child in mild distress. CBC reveals a leukocyte count of 19,000/mm^3. The infant is diagnosed with facial cellulitis and treated with antibiotics but remains febrile for 8 more days of treatment. A repeat CBC reveals a persistent leukocytosis (WBC 30,000/mm^3). Serum immunoglobulin levels are normal. Nitroblue tetrazolium dye reduction test is normal. Analysis of leukocyte cell surface markers by flow cytometry is performed. What does it show?

Flow cytometry shows a **complete absence of cells with β_2-integrins**. **Leukocyte adhesion deficiency** is a rare AR disorder, mainly of neutrophils lacking β_2-**integrins**. Patients often first present with a delayed separation of the umbilical cord and omphalitis (inflammation of the navel). Patients have a h/o recurrent otitis media, aseptic meningitis, and perianal skin lesions and abscesses.

CHAPTER 23

Cell Receptors and Signaling Pathways

INTRODUCTION

Name the different types of cell signaling.	**Autocrine**: self-signaling; released signals act on self.
	Paracrine: short-range signaling; signals are released and act locally on neighboring cells.
	Endocrine: long-range signaling; signal molecules are released into the blood and can act throughout the body.
	Contact-dependent: both the receptor and signaling molecule are membrane bound and require direct contact.
Name the three main families of cell-surface receptors that transmit extracellular signals into the cell.	1. **Ion channel–linked receptor**: opens or closes transiently, allowing ions to diffuse down a gradient 2. **G-protein–linked receptor**: associated with trimeric guanosine 5′-triphosphate (GTP)-binding proteins 3. **Enzyme-linked receptor**: for example, receptor tyrosine kinases
What molecule determines the specific cellular response in a signaling cascade?	Cytosolic portion of a receptor. For example, acetylcholine (ACh) binding to its receptor on the skeletal muscle cell instructs it to contract. However, ACh binding to its receptor on the cardiac myocyte instructs it to relax.
What are the key characteristics of second messenger molecules?	1. Formed in **large quantities** 2. **Rapidly** formed and rapidly deactivated 3. Work as an **amplification signal**

Ca^{2+} is a very common second messenger molecule. Why is it important for cells to maintain very low intracellular [Ca^{2+}]?

The cell becomes more sensitive to very small alterations in Ca^{2+} content, allowing small fluctuations in [Ca^{2+}] to activate signaling pathways.

What methods do cells use to preserve such low intracellular Ca^{2+} levels?

The **Ca^{2+} ATPase pump** and the **Na$^+$/Ca^{2+} antiporter** maintain the low intracellular [Ca^{2+}] by pumping Ca^{2+} out of the cell or, in the case of muscle cells, into the sarcoplasmic reticulum.

Explain how the same ligand may elicit different cellular responses.

Differing receptor subtypes. Although the ligand-binding extracellular portion of the receptor may be the same, in the cytosol, the receptor may be linked to different ion channels or second messengers, resulting in dissimilar effects.

ION CHANNEL–LINKED RECEPTORS

What are two main mechanisms for activating an ion channel–linked receptor?

Ligand-gated or voltage-gated

What determines the direction and rate of ion flow once an ion channel–linked receptor is activated?

Direction: concentration gradient and transmembrane potential of that ion

Rate: number of open channels and the ion concentration gradient across the membrane

What characteristics of an ion channel explain its selectivity?

Size of the ion channel pore, the ionic **charge**, and **electrostatic interactions**

How can a K$^+$ channel be selective against Na$^+$, Cl$^-$, and cesium ions?

Size: cesium ions are too large to fit through the channel pore.

Charge repulsion: K$^+$ channel is lined with negatively charged residues, filtering out Cl$^-$ ions.

Electrostatic interactions: the opening of the K$^+$ channel is lined with carbonyl residues, allowing displacement of the typical water-K$^+$ interaction and passage of dehydrated K$^+$ ions. Hydrated Na$^+$ ions are too small to interact with the carbonyl residues and are therefore too bulky to pass.

Explain how the *N*-methyl-D-aspartate (NMDA) receptor is both voltage-gated and ligand-dependent for activation.

Ligand: glutamate (ligand) and glycine (cofactor) are required for channel opening.

Voltage-gated: membrane depolarization changes the membrane potential, resulting in the removal of the Mg^{2+} ion from the channel pore and permits Na^+ and Ca^{2+} influx and K^+ efflux.

Why does the toxin curare cause flaccid paralysis?

Curare is a **receptor antagonist for nicotinic AChRs**, a ligand-gated ion channel on skeletal muscle cells at the neuromuscular junction (NMJ). It prevents ACh from binding, thereby preventing depolarization and subsequent contraction of myocytes leading to paralysis.

G-PROTEIN–COUPLED RECEPTORS

Describe the cycle of G-protein activation and inactivation. See Figure 23.1.

The heterotrimeric G-protein is composed of the α, β, and γ subunits. It is found as cytosolic proteins or coupled to a receptor.

1. A ligand binds to a G-protein–coupled receptor (GPCR).
2. The α-GDP subunit is phosphorylated. This allows both α and βγ subunits to dissociate from the receptor.
3. Both subunits can act as intracellular signaling molecules.
4. Signaling is terminated when the α subunit, which has guanosine triphosphatase (GTPase) activity, hydrolyzes the guanosine 5′-triphosphate (GTP) to guanosine 5′-diphosphate (GDP).
5. The inactive α-GDP then reassociates with βγ subunits to resume the resting heterotrimeric state.

Illustrated is one of the major signaling pathways. Adenylate cyclase is involved in cyclic adenosine monophosphate (cAMP) and Ca^{2+} amplification, which exerts many physiologic effects.

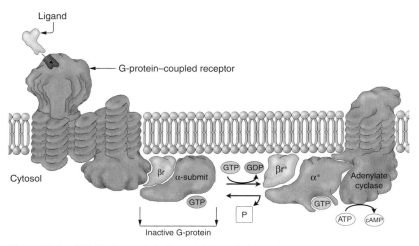

Extracellular space

Ligand

G-protein–coupled receptor

Cytosol

Inactive G-protein

Figure 23.1   GTP-binding protein (G-protein) coupled receptor.

How does the cell respond to such a large variety of signaling responses from just a few different types of ligands that bind GPCRs?

The mammalian genome encodes many different α, β, and γ subunits, allowing extensive variation in the heterotrimeric combination.

Name three main G_α subunit types.

1. G_s (stimulatory)
2. G_i (inhibitory)
3. G_q

Table 23.1   G-protein α Subunit Types

	G_s	G_i	G_q
Types of receptors	β_1, β_2, D_1, H_2, V_2	M_2, α_2, D_2	H_1, α_1, V_1, M_1, M_3
Types of ligands	Adrenaline, glucagon, LH, PTH, ACTH	Somatostatin	Angiotensin, vasopressin, TSH
Function	Stimulates adenylyl cyclase; increases cAMP	Inhibits adenylyl; activates cyclase; decreases cAMP	Activates phospholipase cAMP C; can activate IP_3 or DAG

Abbreviations: α, α-adrenergic; ACTH, adrenocorticotropic hormone; β, β-adrenergic; cAMP, cyclic adenosine monophosphate; D, dopaminergic; DAG, diacylglycerol; H, histaminergic; IP_3, inositol triphosphate; LH, luteinizing hormone; M, muscarinic; PTH, parathyroid hormone; TSH, thyroid-stimulating hormone; V, vasopressin receptors.

How does signaling through the G_q protein lead to mobilization of intracellular calcium stores?

G_q activates phospholipase C, which is responsible for the cleavage of phosphatidylinositol 4, 5 bisphosphate (PIP_2) to generate the second messengers, diacylglycerol (DAG) and inositol triphosphate (IP_3). IP_3 is responsible for intracellular Ca^{2+} mobilization by binding to ligand-gated Ca^{2+} channels located on the ER (IP_3 receptors).

How does this signaling pathway differ from activation of ryanodine receptors?

Ryanodine receptors and IP_3 receptors are both located on the ER and increase intracellular Ca^{2+} levels. IP_3 receptors are ligand-gated, and ryanodine receptors require Ca^{2+} ligands and are also activated by the initial increase in Ca^{2+} causing membrane depolarization.

What determines the duration of G-protein–coupled receptor signaling?

The **rate of GTP hydrolysis** by GTPases, which leads to α subunit inactivation

ENZYME-LINKED RECEPTORS

Name the five known classes of enzyme-linked receptors.

1. Receptor tyrosine kinases
2. Tyrosine kinase–associated receptors
3. Receptor serine/threonine kinases
4. Transmembrane guanylyl cyclases
5. Histidine kinase–associated receptors

Explain how a receptor tyrosine kinase is activated.

Ligand binding induces a **conformational change** in the receptor, **receptor dimerization**, and **transphosphorylation of tyrosine residues** on the cytoplasmic tail.

How do activated tyrosine kinase receptors recruit specific signaling proteins to their cytosolic tails?

Autophosphorylation of tyrosine residues on the receptor creates docking sites for proteins containing Src-homology 2 (Sh2) domains and phosphotyrosine binding (PTB) domains.

Describe the signaling cascade induced by receptor tyrosine kinases that results in mitogen-activated protein (MAP) kinase activation and phosphorylation of transcription factors. See Figure 23.2.

Growth factor binding to a tyrosine kinase receptor leads to phosphorylation of the receptor itself and activation of Ras. Ras activates the serine/threonine kinase Raf, which phosphorylates and activates MEK (MAP kinase/ERK kinase). MEK then phosphorylates extracellular signal-regulated kinase (ERK). Activated ERK phosphorylates many downstream kinases and also translocates to the nucleus to phosphorylate transcription factors.

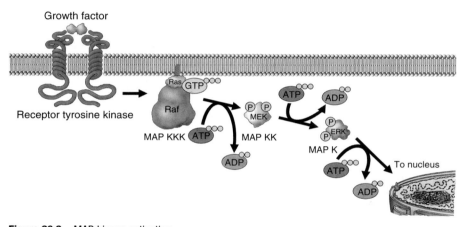

Figure 23.2   MAP kinase activation.

How are signals from receptor tyrosine kinases turned off?

The receptors are endocytosed by **receptor-mediated endocytosis** to stop the signaling.

What are some examples of ligands that bind to receptor tyrosine kinases?

FGF (fibroblast growth factor)

EGF (epidermal growth factor)

PDGF (platelet-derived growth factor)

VEGF (vascular endothelial growth factor)

Provide an example of how integrin-mediated intracellular signaling differs from conventional signaling receptors.

Signaling by integrins can provide **localized responses**. For example, axon guidance and pathfinding is partially mediated by the interaction of integrins on the growing axon tip (the growth cone) and the extracellular matrix. Local adhesive signaling influences the response of growth cones to attractive or repellent environmental cues during both development and regeneration.

STEROID RECEPTORS

What class of receptors do steroid receptors belong to?

Nuclear receptor superfamily. They are ligand-gated proteins that bind DNA and function to regulate gene expression.

Provide some examples of ligands for steroid receptors.

Extracellular, hydrophobic signaling molecules (eg, thyroid hormone, steroid hormone, retinoids, and vitamin D) or intracellular metabolites

Why do the hormones testosterone and estrogen make good ligands for steroid receptors?

They are **hydrophobic**, permitting diffusion through the plasma membrane.

Why does signal transduction through steroid receptors require a longer response time compared to voltage-gated receptors?

Activated steroid receptors translocate to the nucleus where they act as transcription factors to **mediate transcription**. Unlike the instantaneous response of a voltage-gated receptor, gene expression may take hours before a response is detectable.

Why do steroid receptor responses persist for a longer duration?

Even after ligand-receptor dissociation, the cellular response persists until the protein is degraded or transcription is downregulated.

What are heat-shock proteins (hsp)?

Molecular **chaperones** that mediate protein folding

What is the significance of being activated at elevated temperatures?

Heat tends to denature proteins. Thus, hsp synthesis is typically increased in elevated temperatures.

What is the role of hsp in intracellular-steroid receptor signaling?	When inactive, steroid receptors are bound to heat-shock proteins in a ligand-friendly conformation prohibiting nuclear translocation. Upon ligand binding, the receptor undergoes conformational change exposing the DNA binding domain and separating from the hsp.
How does the thyroid hormone receptor lead to both, activation and repression of the same target gene?	Without its ligand, the thyroid hormone receptor is constitutively bound to hormone response elements (HREs) on DNA and represses gene transcription. In the presence of thyroid hormone, the ligand-receptor complex activates gene transcription.
Explain how steroid receptor isoforms can lead to hormone concentration–dependent transcription.	Isoforms vary in their ligand affinity, allowing those with stronger ligand affinity to synthesize proteins during lower concentrations of hormone.

CLINICAL CORRELATES AND VIGNETTES

How does diazepam, a benzodiazepine, produce its anxiolytic effect?

Benzodiazepines **increase the affinity of the GABA$_A$ receptor** for its ligand, GABA. GABA is the major CNS inhibitory neurotransmitter and activating this ligand-gated ion channel increases Cl^- influx and membrane hyperpolarization.

Morphine, an opioid-receptor agonist, is a well-known analgesic with multiple side effects. These side effects include respiratory depression, vomiting, and constipation. How can one drug cause multiple effects throughout the body?

Different receptor subtypes and their varied **distribution** in the body can lead to multiple effects. Morphine selectively binds to μ-opioid receptors, but at higher concentrations, may also bind to κ- and δ-opioid receptors. The analgesic effect of morphine is due to ligand binding of μ-opioid receptors in the CNS, thus altering neuronal pain pathways. The μ-opioid receptor is also located in the medullary respiratory control center and the gastrointestinal tract leading to many other side effects.

How does the cholera toxin cause diarrhea?

Cholera toxin is an **ADP-ribosylating toxin**. ADP ribosylation of the α_s inactivates its GTPase activity. The constituitively active α_s activates adenylyl cyclase, elevating cAMP levels. In the small intestine, high levels of cAMP increase the secretion of water, Na^+, K^+ Cl^-, and HCO_3^{3-} into the lumen.

How does estrogen-induced gap junction upregulation in the uterus aid the initiation of labor?

During most of pregnancy, the uterine cells contain few gap junctions, resulting in weak, uncoordinated contractions. Gap junction upregulation late in pregnancy enables rapid action potential spread throughout the uterine smooth muscle and synchronizes smooth muscle contractions to generate a larger force.

Spironolactone acts as a diuretic by inhibiting aldosterone-induced transcription of Na^+/K^+ ATPase and Na^+ channels at the distal nephron. Explain how spironolactone inhibits aldosterone. How does aldosterone alter transcription?

Spironolactone is a competitive inhibitor of the cytosolic aldosterone receptor located in the distal tubule and collecting duct of the kidneys. Aldosterone-receptor interaction allows translocation to the nucleus and transcriptional regulation.

A 4 mo infant p/w a nonproductive cough, fever, and difficulty feeding for 3 weeks. Over the last 3 days, the cough became so severe that the infant was unable to catch his breath and turned blue while coughing. On exam, the infant appears very agitated and dehydrated. Auscultation of the chest reveals diffuse wheezes and rales and a respiratory rate of 50 after a coughing paroxysm. A CXR reveals perihilar infiltrates and patchy atelectasis. The WBC count is 30,000/mm^3 with an 80% lymphocytosis. What would a nasopharyngeal swab show?

Bordetella pertussis can be cultured from the nasopharynx. Pertussis is highly contagious and is characterized by severe bronchitis. The onset of pertussis or the **"whooping cough"** is insidious. A paroxysmal cough characterized by 10 to 30 forceful coughs and ending with a loud inspiration is a hallmark. There is usually a lymphocytosis of 70% to 80%. The pertussis toxin catalyzes the ADP ribosylation of the G-protein, blocking inhibition of adenylate cyclase by G_i. Erythromycin is the antibiotic of choice.

A 35 yo obese F of short stature and a round face p/w shortening of the fourth and fifth metacarpal bones and mental retardation. What is the mutation in her syndrome?

Albright hereditary osteodystrophy, also known as **pseudohypoparathyroidism**, is due to a mutation in the parathyroid hormone (PTH) receptor on the end organs. It is an inactivating mutation in the α subunit of the G_s protein. Although there are elevated amounts of PTH in the serum, the patient is persistently hypocalcemic and hyperphosphatemic.

260 Deja Review: Histology & Cell Biology

A 45 yo F c/o dry mouth and muscle weakness with difficulty rising from chairs and climbing stairs. Her symptoms are worse in the mornings but improve during the day and with exercise. On neurologic exam, she has proximal lower extremity weakness and loss of b/l knee jerks. Her extraocular muscles are intact. A repetitive nerve stimulation examination reveals an incremental response of the compound muscle action potentials. What is this woman suffering from?

Eaton-Lambert syndrome manifests with hip-girdle weakness. An autoantibody directed against the presynaptic voltage-gated Ca^{2+} channels on the nerve membranes slows the entry of Ca^{2+} into the presynaptic terminal. With repetitive depolarizations, enough Ca^{2+} accumulates allowing eventual vesicular release of ACh and improves muscle strength. This explains the incremental increase in amplitude of muscle action potential with repetitive stimulation.

Suggested Readings

Alberts J, Lewis R, Roberts W, eds. *Molecular Biology of the Cell.* 4th ed. New York, NY: Garland Science; 2002.

Barrett KE, Barman SM, Boitano S, Brooks H. *Ganong's Review of Medical Physiology.* 23rd ed. New York, NY: McGraw- Hill; 2010.

Fawcett DW, Jensh, RP. *Concise Histology.* New York, NY: Chapman and Hall; 1997.

Gartner LP, Hiatt JL. *Color Textbook of Histology.* Philadelphia, PA: W. B. Saunders Co; 1997.

Le T, Takiar V. *First Aid Cases for the USMLE Step 1.* 2nd ed. New York, NY: McGraw Hill; 2009.

Lilly LS, ed. *Pathophysiology of Heart Disease.* 3rd ed. Philadelphia, PA: Lippincott Williams & Wilkins; 2003.

Mescher AL. *Junqueira's Basic Histology: Text and Atlas.* 12th ed. New York, NY: McGraw- Hill; 2010.

Sternberg SS, ed. *Histology for Pathologists.* 2nd ed. Philadelphia, PA: Lippincott-Raven; 1997.

Wilson FJ, Kestenbaum MG, Gibney JA, Matta S. *Histology Image Review.* Norwalk, CT: Appleton & Lange; 1997.

Abbreviations

[ ] denotes concentration
ACh acetylcholine
AChR acetylcholine receptors
ACTH adrenocorticotropic hormone
AD autosomal dominant
ADH antidiuretic hormone
ADP adenosine diphosphate
ALT alanine aminotransferase
ANP atrial natriuretic peptide
APCs antigen presenting cells
AR autosomal recessive
AST aspartate aminotransferase
ATP adenosine triphosphate
ATPase adenosine triphosphatase
b/l bilateral
BBB blood-brain barrier
BP blood pressure
bpm beats per minute
BRBPR bright red blood per rectum
c/o complains of
CABG coronary artery bypass grafting
cAMP cyclic adenosine monophosphate
CBC complete blood cell count
CD collecting duct
cDNA complementary DNA
cm centimeter
CML chronic myeloid leukemia
CN cranial nerve
CNS central nervous system
CO carbon monoxide
CO_2 carbon dioxide
CP chest pain
CRH corticotropin-releasing hormone
CSF cerebrospinal fluid
CT cat scan
CXR chest X-ray
DAG diacylglycerol
DCT distal convoluted tubule
DES diethylstilbestrol
DHEAS dehydroepiandrosterone sulfate
DM diabetes mellitus
DNA Deoxyribonucleic acid
ECL enterochromaffin-like
ED emergency department
EDS Ehlers-Danlos syndrome
EDTA ethylene diamine tetra acetic acid
EGF epidermal growth factor
EKG electrocardiogram
ELIZA enzyme-linked immunosorbent
assay
ER endoplasmic reticulum
ERCP endoscopic retrograde
  cholangiopancreatography
F female
FHx family history
FSH follicle-stimulating hormone
GABA gamma-aminobutyric acid
GDP guanosine 5′-diphosphate
GERD gastroesophageal reflux disease
GH growth hormone
GnRH gonadotropin-releasing hormone
GPCR G-protein–coupled receptors
GTP guanosine 5′-triphosphate
h/o history of
hCS human chorionic
  somatomammotropin
HGP Human Genome Project
HIV human immunodeficiency virus
hnRNA heterogeneous nuclear RNA
HR heart rate
HTN hypertension
ICU intensive care unit
IgA immunoglobulin A
IgE immunoglobulin E
IGF insulin-like growth factor
IGF-1 insulin-like growth factor-1
IP_3 inositol triphosphate
LDH lactate dehydrogenase

LDL low-density lipoprotein
LH luteinizing hormone
LLQ left lower quadrant
M male
M-6-P mannose-6-phosphate
MAP mitogen activated protein
MEK MAP kinase/ERK kinase
MI myocardial infarction
min minute(s)
MIS müllerian inhibiting substance
mo month
mo month old
mRNA messenger RNA
MSH mismatch repair enzymes
mtDNA mitochondrial DNA
N/V nausea and vomiting
NIS Na+/I– symporters
nm nanometer
NMDA N-methyl-D-aspartate
NMJ neuromuscular junction
NSAIDs nonsteroidal anti-inflammatory
  drugs
NTD neural tube defect
o/w otherwise
p/w presents with
PCP primary care physician
PCR polymerase chain reaction
PE physical exam
PIP$_2$ phosphatidylinositol 4,
  5 bisphosphate

PMHx past medical history
PNS peripheral nervous system
PPI proton pump inhibitors
PRL prolactin
PTB phospho-tyrosine binding
PTH parathyroid hormone
RBC red blood cells
RER rough endoplasmic reticulum
rRNA ribosomal RNA
RT-PCR reverse transcriptase-PCR
RUQ right upper quadrant
SDS sodium dodecyl sulfate
SER smooth endoplasmic reticulum
Sh2 Src-homology 2
SOB shortness of breath
SR sarcoplasmic reticulum
SRP signal recognition particle
SSBP single-strand DNA binding protein
SSTR simple sequence tandem repeats
TB tuberculosis
tRNA transfer RNA
TSH thyroid-stimulating hormone
US ultrasound
VNTR variable number of tandem
  repeats
WBC white blood cells
x-ray radiograph
yo year-old

Index

Page numbers followed by f or t indicate figures or tables, respectively.